Health and Exclusion

While practices and policies of exclusion have always characterised health care systems and the professional groups who work with them, recent changes to the NHS, as well as wider, more global structural changes, have increased the focus on exclusion as a key theme in both health care and health work. *Health and Exclusion* addresses exclusion from a number of informing perspectives in terms of health care policy and practice.

In addition to documenting examples of exclusion in the health services, the book discusses the impact of poverty on the health of low-income households with children; the contribution of health promotion strategies to maintaining exclusion and marginalisation; exclusion in maternity care; the social exclusion of those with mental health problems and the role of doctors and nurses in this process; the silencing of the patient's voice in medical encounters; and the exclusion experienced by older people using health services. Other themes covered include resistance to exclusion through strategies of empowerment and the challenges to professional autonomy and power mounted by 'managerialism'.

Health and Exclusion challenges New Labour's 'third way' and emphasises the wider framework for understanding exclusion in a health care context. It is essential reading for health professionals and students of social policy and sociology.

Michael Purdy is Lecturer in Nursing at the University of Sheffield and **David Banks** is Senior Lecturer at the School of Health, University of Teesside.

Health and Exclusion

Policy and practice in health provision

Edited by Michael Purdy and David Banks

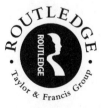

London and New York

SMC

First published 1999
by Routledge
11 New Fetter Lane, London EC4P 4EE

Simultaneously published in the USA and Canada
by Routledge
29 West 35th Street, New York, NY 10001

Routledge is an imprint of the Taylor & Francis Group   360 PuR

© 1999 Selection and editorial matter, Michael Purdy and
David Banks; individual chapters, the contributors

Typeset in Sabon by Routledge
Printed and bound in Great Britain by St Edmundsbury Press,
Bury St Edmunds, Suffolk

British Library Cataloguing in Publication Data
A catalogue record for this book is available from the British Library

Library of Congress Cataloging in Publication Data
Health and exclusion: policy and practice in health provision /
Edited by Michael Purdy and David Banks.
    Includes bibliographical references and index.
    1. Health services accessibility – Great Britain.
    2. Discrimination in medical care – Great Britain.
    3. Medical care – utilisation – Great Britain.
    4. Medical care – social aspects – Great Britain.
    5. Poor – medical care – Great Britain.
    I. Purdy, Michael, 1953– . II. Banks, David, 1956– .
    RA418.3.G7H425   1999   98-51639
    CIP

ISBN 0–415–18016–3 (hbk)
ISBN 0–415–18017–1 (pbk)

Contents

vi *Contents*

Contributors

David Banks is a Senior Lecturer in the School of Health at the University of Teesside. From a background in mental health nursing he has worked in nurse education for the last ten years. His present research and writing interests include published and ongoing work on communication, ethnicity and professional identity.

Clare Blackburn is a Senior Research Fellow in the Department of Applied Social Studies at the University of Warwick. Her research is concerned with poverty and the health of households with children and the implications of this research for the practice of health practitioners.

John Clarke is Professor of Social Policy at the Open University. His most recent work concerns the impact of managerialism on social welfare. He is the co-author, with Janet Newman, of *The Managerial State: power, politics and ideology in the remaking of social welfare* (Sage 1997).

Sue Davies is a Lecturer in Nursing in the Department of Gerontological and Continuing Care Nursing at the University of Sheffield. Current research includes an international comparison of relatives' experiences of nursing home entry in collaboration with colleagues in Sweden and Australia.

Nick J. Fox is a Senior Lecturer in Sociology at the University of Sheffield. He is the author of *The Social Meaning of Surgery* (Open University Press 1992) and *Postmodernism, Sociology and Health* (Open University Press 1993), and numerous journal articles on postmodernism.

Mavis Kirkham is Professor of Midwifery at the University of Sheffield. She has twenty-five years' experience of midwifery practice and research.

Brian D. Loader is currently Co-Director of the Community Informatics & Applications Unit (CIRA) based at the University of Teesside. He is General Editor of the international journal *Information, Communication and Society* (Routledge), and his recent publications include *The Governance of Cyberspace* (Routledge 1997) and *Cyberspace Divide* (Routledge 1998).

Peter Alan Morrall is a Senior Lecturer in Health and Sociology at the University of Leeds. With twenty-five years' experience of working, teaching and researching in the field of psychiatric disorder, he is viewed as an 'internal critic' of the mental health system and what he describes as the 'self-serving doctrines' of the psychiatric professionals. He has recently published *Mental Health Nursing and Social Control* (Whurr 1998).

Michael Purdy is a Lecturer in Nursing at the University of Sheffield. His research and writing interests are in the sociology and politics of health, with a particular concern for the role of health promotion and public health strategies and practices as instruments of social regulation.

Alan Walker is Professor of Social Policy at the University of Sheffield. He has been researching and writing on the issues of poverty, social exclusion and ageing for many years. Recent books include *Britain Divided* (1997), *Ageing Europe* (1998) and *The Social Quality of Europe* (1998).

Preface

This book is about social exclusion and health, about the ways in which certain individuals, groups, classes and communities today experience inequality and disadvantage in either the health care they receive, or the health work they perform. The intention has been to present a sample of the policies and practices of exclusion currently experienced by patients and users of the health services in the United Kingdom, and by nurses and other health professionals providing these services. We acknowledge that, in offering a sample of exclusion in health care and health work, other significant sites of exclusion have been omitted.

Despite its common use, the term 'social exclusion' is by no means a straightforward concept, and many of the contributors to this volume draw attention to its complexity. In particular the notion of exclusion as a single and simple binary process is rejected and with it the belief that the excluded can be identified as a homogeneous group, such as an 'underclass', easily distinguishable at the margins of society. Contemporary exclusion is a more fluid process, with individuals, families and communities often moving in and out of an excluded or marginalised status. However, this is not to deny a multiplier effect whereby disadvantage and exclusion in one area of social experience combine with other forces to produce multiple disadvantage. Discussions of social exclusion need to be sensitive to significant differences in the experience of exclusion within a population. Full recognition must be given to the divided and unequal social environment which mediates these experiences. In short, and as Levitas (1996) argues, the concept of social exclusion should not be permitted to obscure the fundamental social class divisions which continue to structure life chances in our society.

Whilst a range of work has been published on the other components of the welfare state (see for example Loney *et al.* 1991,

Gladstone 1995), this text fills a gap in the literature by explicitly addressing social exclusion from the perspective of health and health care. It should appeal to a wide readership, insofar as the collection is intended both to provide a reader for health and social science students concerned with making sense of social exclusion, and to offer new and original contributions to the contemporary policy debate regarding social exclusion.

The collection is timely, for two reasons. First, because the experience of exclusion in Britain has increased enormously during the last twenty years, and second because the issues of social exclusion and inequality are once again on the political agenda in this country following the election of a Labour government in May 1997. It is these two 'facts', of the increasing polarisation of British society and the potential for central government action to challenge exclusion, that provide the rationale for this book. The question of the extent to which the election to office of New Labour, with its commitment to a new NHS (DOH 1997), will significantly challenge inequalities and exclusion in the field of health is an open one, and is addressed by many of the contributors to this volume. It is fair to say that social policy analysis has tended to steer clear of the health debate, which has largely been dominated by the previous government's policy focus on managerialism and the technicalities of rationing health care provision.

This book is very much concerned with health and exclusion in the 1990s. However, if contemporary forms of social exclusion are the focus, a central theme of the collection is that these examples of exclusion in the health field cannot be understood without situating them both historically and in relation to wider contemporary patterns and processes of social and economic change, political ideology and professional interests. In this way 'continuities' and 'discontinuities' in relations of exclusion can be identified.

We *do not* claim to have an overarching theoretical paradigm with which to address questions of exclusion in health and health care. Contributors have approached the subject from a number of different perspectives. In this way the collection goes some way to reflecting the richness and diversity of debate which is emerging in the fields of health theory, policy, practice and experience.

Michael Purdy
David Banks
March 1999

References

Department of Health (DOH) (1997) *The New NHS: Modern, Dependable*, London: The Stationery Office.

Gladstone, D. (ed.) (1995) *British Social Welfare: Past, Present and Future*, London: UCL Press.

Levitas, R. (1996) 'The concept of social exclusion and the new Durkheimian hegemony', *Critical Social Policy* 16, 46: 5–20.

Loney, M., Bocock, R., Clarke, J., Cochrane, A., Graham, P. and Wilson, M. (eds) (1991) *The State or the Market: Politics and Welfare in Contemporary Britain*, 2nd edition, London: Sage.

1 Tracing continuity and diversity in health and exclusion

Michael Purdy and David Banks

The historical context

The National Health Service (NHS) recently celebrated its fiftieth anniversary, and it seems fitting that its promise of equity in health care should be assessed. The distance that the NHS has travelled in this period is paralleled by the development of the Labour party from a government committed to ideals of social justice in 1948 to one which, in 1998, declared its intention of ending inequality and combating social exclusion. However, it is too easy simply to interpret the NHS and the changes it has experienced over the last fifty years in terms of party politics and contrasting ideologies of 'collectivism' and 'individualism'.

A seductive history of the NHS would have us believe that its aspirations to alleviate the inequalities of health which confronted it at its birth in 1948 were destroyed in the late 1970s as a Tory government embarked on the dismantling of the 'welfare state' and the principles of social justice that it embraced. The end of the 'consensus' on state welfarism which the New Right policies of Margaret Thatcher are seen to signify unfortunately hides the bitter truth that, long before the international economic crisis of the 1970s and the reviews of state welfare expenditure of the 1980s, the British welfare state (including the NHS) was regularly and systematically generating inequalities of income, health and life chances. This capacity to exclude had its roots in the conditions of compromise upon which the welfare state depended for its very existence.

The notion that the post-war welfare state established universal welfare rights must be rejected as a myth. For welfare has been available only to those *recognised* as citizens in the first place (Cochrane 1993). Social divisions of class, race and gender have been reproduced in people's experiences of, and unequal access to, welfare provision (Williams 1993, Baldwin and Falkingham 1994, O'Brien and Penna 1998). These inequalities and the social exclusion they permit have been tolerated by Labour and Conservative governments alike.

The political consensus between Tory and Labour governments over state welfare between 1948 and the late 1970s can therefore be read as a consensus as much over exclusion as over achieving greater social justice. In the field of health, 'universal' access to health care was never more than a promise, inequalities in health persisted, with both Labour and Conservative administrations consistently failing to tackle them directly (Allsop 1995), and an 'inverse care law' became the norm.

Evidence of the salience of social divisions such as that of 'social class' to people's experience of health and of health services throughout the lifetime of the NHS is not hard to find. Reporting in 1979, the Black Report (Townsend and Davidson 1982) pointed to an inverse relationship between social class and mortality and 'provided evidence of a persistent class gradient in mortality, despite the improvements experienced by all groups in the post-war period' (Bury 1997: 60). Subsequent reports (for example, Whitehead 1992, Phillimore *et al.* 1994, Drever and Whitehead 1997, Richardson and Reid 1997, Acheson 1998, Shaw *et al.* 1998) have confirmed the continued widening of inequalities in health since 1979. In addition to social class, inequalities in morbidity and mortality rates have been shown to exist along other social dimensions in the United Kingdom, including those of gender, geographical location and ethnic background (DOH 1995).

The continued existence of inequalities and exclusion in health raises the question of the extent to which the welfare state and the NHS can be judged to be a success or to have failed. To say that the welfare state has failed because it hasn't delivered 'equality' (Le Grand 1982) may be to miss the point that equalisation and redistribution were never its intention (Hindess 1987). It was never established as a means to redistribute from the rich to the poor, lacking as it did any 'principle of targeting' and including 'the middle classes for the first time as major beneficiaries of welfare services' (Glennerster 1990). Consequently, social and welfare policies should perhaps be judged on the basis of the equality of opportunity and access which they deliver. In these terms a basis exists (i) for recognising *both* success and failure of the NHS (for example, in offering greater access to the population as a whole compared to pre-1948, whilst still excluding certain groups from full and equal access to services); (ii) for criticising the excesses of Tory New Right policies and ideology in the field of health and welfare (i.e. in restricting and reducing access further since 1979); (iii) for identifying the sorts of interventions necessary to increase access and reduce exclusion in health and health care (e.g. central government policies on housing, transport, employment, education and income); and (iv) for questioning the direction of New Labour policies, which in continuing to restructure welfare and expand the mixed economy of welfare without a policy of income redistribution (through income tax rather than means tested and targeted benefits), will fail to increase opportunities for access or reduce the risks of exclusion.

The contemporary context

Contemporary patterns of exclusion in the United Kingdom bear witness to the impact of global economic and technological change insofar as international rather than purely domestic forces have called into question the ability of the British state to sustain its post-war commitments to state welfarism.

Post-Fordism provides the broadest context for situating recent challenges to state welfarism, associated policy developments and practices of exclusion. It refers to a shift in social, cultural and economic structures and relationships from their relatively stable configuration under conditions of advanced capitalism established after the end of the Second World War and upon which the welfare state was built. The post-war configuration of Fordism constituted a 'distinctive period of economic growth', characterised by the harnessing of economic activity to the large-scale mass production of standardised goods for mass markets under the direction of hierarchical systems of centralised management and control; 'Fordism is summarized as the age of "intensive accumulation" with "monopolistic regulation" of the economy' (Amin 1994: 9).

The stability of Fordism as a regime of accumulation, social regulation and reproduction ruptured during the 1970s as the international capitalist order moved into a state of structural crisis, with the stagnation of the international economy. This crisis effectively applied the brake to 'the unimpeded expansion of welfare services' by western governments (Berridge and Webster 1993). The post-war consensus on welfare policy was shattered, and after 1974 British governments of both major political parties conducted a reappraisal of policy and searched for economies.

Post-Fordism signifies a period of transition in which future development appears to require different economic, social and political norms. 'Localism' and 'adaptability' are key features of the new era, and the ability of the state to manage economic activity in this period is severely compromised. The bureaucracy of a centralised state management structure thwarts the need for adaptability and flexibility, and increasing 'globalisation' of capital accumulation, investment patterns and market activity raises serious doubts as to the viability of the 'nation state' as the site for managing future regimes of accumulation (Alcock 1996). The global economic 'web' replaces hierarchical systems of centralised control with dispersed trans-global networks, which permit subnational local sites to by-pass national state structures, traverse national boundaries and link directly with any other site in the world.

The inability of the nation state to manage the emerging regime of accumulation is not, however, the sole point of its weakness following the crisis of Fordism. Related to this is the challenge that post-Fordism mounts to its status as the principal site of social regulation. Under conditions of Fordist accumulation, the Keynesian state was able to finance and expand the welfare state, maintaining an apparatus of social regulation through its sponsorship of a partnership between labour and capital. Following Fordism the state is no longer able to sustain this regulatory role. Now Western governments are forced to direct their attention towards restructuring their interventionist activities with a view to both containing costs and attracting global investment through the suppression of welfare costs. Social policy is becoming global as national policies are increasingly determined by 'global economic competition' and the 'locus of key policy decisions' shifts from national governments to global banking organisations (Deacon 1997).

Out of this crisis in welfare and the global economic restructuring that provides its widest context, new forms of 'governance' are beginning to emerge (see, for example, Rhodes 1997) and debate develops over the likely shape of a 'post-Fordist welfare state' (e.g. Burrows and Loader 1994) and 'postmodern' forms of welfare (e.g. Carter 1998).

Underpinning the new forms of governance is a discourse of 'managerialism', which Clarke and Newman (1997) identify as central to the remaking of the welfare state, signalling the emergence of what they call 'the managerial state', and the transformation of state power into new organisational forms. Specifically, this has involved the displacement of 'bureaucratic administration' and 'professionalism' as the 'modes of connection' upon which the welfare state has rested since 1948. Far from the state being 'rolled back', the period of restructuring is seen to have involved 'a "rolling out" of state power but in new and dispersed forms' (ibid: 30), coordinated through the ideology and practices of 'managerialism'.

In his contribution to this volume, Clarke (Chapter 3) highlights the significance for contemporary patterns of exclusion in health of these wider processes of change by examining the relationship between recent changes in the organisation of health services and changes in the form and role of the state in social welfare. The 'managerialisation' of state welfare is shown to have led to 'perverse consequences' for the welfare of the public as state services are put on a more 'businesslike' footing. The pursuit of economy and efficiency in the provision of publicly funded services, for example, involves the more explicit use of such strategies as 'rationing' and 'targeting' in the deployment of health and welfare services. In this process, organisational efficiency can be increased by 'externalising' the costs of welfare, that is by transferring the costs to other (non-state) organisations, services or sectors. The efficient and economic use of state-sponsored health and welfare services may therefore be bought at the price of a deterioration in the public health of those sections of the population whose health and welfare needs are no longer recognised to be 'the business' of the state.

The question of the effects of organisational change on exclusion in health is also raised by Loader (Chapter 10), who focuses on the impact of new 'informational and communications technologies' on health care organisation. Loader argues that we are witnessing the emergence of a new form of health care organisation in which 'vertically integrated command and control structures' are being replaced by an organisational control paradigm which relies on 'self regulation and decentralised autonomous control strategies'. He refers to these new forms of health care organisation as *'informational health networks'*. The government's new NHS (DOH 1997), for example, comprises 'a plurality of nodal points in the form of PCGs, Health Authorities, NHS Trusts, local authorities, and Regional and National Health Authorities', in which responsibility for the management of health is increasingly devolved to individuals themselves through improved direct access to home-based advice and information on 'health, illness and the NHS'. Loader emphasises that, whilst 'informational health networks' may be compatible with the principle of a comprehensive and universal health service, and may appear to hold out the prospect of individuals gaining more control over their bodies and health, a danger exists that the 'constellation of power relationships in the network' may act to exclude sections of the community. In short, not everyone will be able to be members of an 'informational health network' due to the constraints and barriers imposed by their social circumstances.

Clarke and Loader draw our attention to the fact that wider processes of social, economic and technological change and the new emergent forms of welfarism that accompany them are likely to contain *both* opportunities for individual empowerment and possibilities for extending and deepening contemporary patterns of exclusion in health.

Welfare restructuring and exclusion in health and health care

The crisis of confidence in the ability of the state to fund and effectively manage universal provision of welfare has involved a process of 'welfare restructuring' and the development of a 'mixed economy of welfare' in which the state redefines its role (Johnson 1990). The emphasis has been on 'welfare pluralism', with the state 'retaining a key role as a guarantor of welfare rights, a regulator of standards and a provider of resources' (Kendall and Moon 1994: 163) and increasingly assuming a 'residual' role as provider of welfare services. In the health field, the NHS has experienced radical structural change with the introduction of an 'internal market' and the establishing of 'consumerism' at the heart of its policy and practice (Butler 1992, Baggott 1994, Ranade 1994, Klein 1995).

Welfare restructuring has resulted in a shift in the balance within the United Kingdom's 'welfare regime' between the state, private, voluntary and informal care sectors. Thus, throughout the 1980s, government sought to shift the burden of responsibility for community care from the state to non-statutory organisations and to the community itself. This shift has had serious repercussions for patterns of exclusion in health.

A discourse of 'consumerism' has been central to the Tory government's reform of community care, with the benefit of increased individual choice held up as the pay-off. Indeed, consumerism has emerged as a powerful means for redefining the welfare rights of the individual, reconstituting these rights in terms of a market relationship rather than in terms of universal rights of citizenship. The question posed by consumerism is: can everyone enjoy consumer rights under a reconstructed welfare state? Clearly, the answer is no. For the very individualism in which consumerism is couched hides the fact that 'social relations shape the experience of consuming' (Edgell and Hetherington 1996). In other words, not everyone is able to be a consumer. Some are excluded from this possibility, since the benefits of consumerism, in the form of increased choice and power, are perhaps available only to those who have the resources to 'buy themselves out of public systems' (Clarke 1996). In these terms, the ideology of consumerism and the health and welfare practices that it has encouraged generate new social divisions and exclusions. Baldock and Ungerson (1996), for example, identify ways in which the 'new community care' requires that people change their expectations and behaviour in order to benefit from the new arrangements. Specifically, older people are confronted with a radically different mixed economy of community care which challenges the values and assumptions of a lifetime. Faced with uncertain and confusing 'conditions of consumption', some are unable to become consumers insofar as they are unable to change (collectivist) values and assumptions that have been fundamental to the ways in which they have lived their lives. As such, they are ill-equipped to deal with a system of care in the community which denies them the services and support that their previous experiences of state welfarism had led them reasonably to expect, and which now calls on them to exercise consumer choice.

Exercising consumer choice presupposes that real choices exist which the consumer is free to choose. Unfortunately, this has not been the experience of older people since the National Health Service and Community Care Act of 1990 'residualised' the provision of public services and opened up 'choice' in an expanded 'mixed economy' of community care. For, as Walker (1993, 1997) has argued, far from enjoying increased choice, the experience of many older people of the market of community care has been that they have no choice at all. Indeed, 'perverse incentives' have operated to produce an '*over*-supply of residential care places' together with a 'tighter rationing of home care', the outcome of which is that 'a significant proportion of older people in private residential homes, perhaps as much as one-half, do not need to occupy residential places on the basis of disability' (1997: 185). In this situation older people are excluded from the decision-making process over the most appropriate care to meet their needs. Far from being a genuine attempt to improve the quality of community care and meet the needs of older people and their carers, the community care reforms are a response to economic and ideological imperatives.

The increasing dependency of older people forms the focus of Walker's contribution to this volume (Chapter 9), which examines 'the role of health services in creating and reinforcing exclusion among older people'. Walker outlines the pivotal role that health professionals have played in constructing dependency in old age through the adoption of a medical or disease model of health combined with wider social attitudes of ageism. The negative consequences for older people include a tendency for them to be regarded as a homogeneous group, for their treatment and social care to be dominated by an institutional approach, and for age discrimination to operate in the provision of screening and other preventive services. The exclusion and disempowerment experienced by many older people and their family carers since the formation of the NHS has been reinforced by the 'marketisation of health and social care' during the last twenty years. Walker argues that the 'consumerist' model of participation and choice offered to older people is clearly inadequate to their needs, and that the only way in which their influence over service provision can be assured is if 'frail and vulnerable' service users 'are guaranteed a "voice" in the organisation and management of services'. Whilst formidable obstacles exist to the 'inclusion and empowerment of older people', including the professionalisation process itself, Walker discusses a number of steps which are necessary to overcoming barriers to user-participation and concludes his chapter by identifying eight key principles for developing more empowering approaches in the practice of health and social care workers. In emphasising that the exclusion and dependency experienced by many older people is socially constructed and related to the demands of a wider political and economic context, Walker points to the possibility of reducing the dependency and exclusion of older people and their family carers in the health arena.

The restructuring process of post-Fordism may involve the abandonment of the universal and collectivist principles found in the Fordist 'regime of accumulation' and supportive 'mode of regulation', with increasing social exclusion, polarisation and marginalisation signifying the 'new order'. Certainly, the current transitionary phase is characterised by 'a tendency towards greater not less economic and social inequality' (Allen 1992) as social programmes are subordinated to the economic priorities of 'innovation and competition' (Mayer 1994). Welfare provision may become increasingly targeted, with 'a scaling down and reorientation of welfare services towards the "economically active" groups in society'

(Amin 1994). Having said this, the crisis of the welfare state cannot satisfactorily be reduced to a crisis of Fordism. Each may have its own dynamic. The form and direction of the restructuring process itself is neither predetermined or inevitable. Different routes out of Fordism are possible and can be pursued.

Whilst all European states since the 1970s have been faced with the need to examine closely their public expenditure and restructure their provision of welfare services (including health) accordingly, British restructuring has resulted in greater inequalities between rich and poor than in any other European country (Walker and Walker 1997). What singled out UK restructuring, and the unparalleled growth in poverty and social exclusion that it generated, were the political and ideological discourses through which it was articulated. The New Right ideology of Thatcherism generated a massive increase in social exclusion, marginalisation and social polarisation (Gamble 1994). And the 'two nations' situation that resulted was reproduced in the health field in both the extension of established patterns of exclusion and the emergence of new ones. Existing inequalities in health between the richest and poorest groups in Britain continued to widen throughout the Thatcher and Major administrations (Benzeval 1997), as government policies of economic and welfare reform reduced the provision of welfare support and generated increased poverty which impacted on many of the 'precursors' for health, such as income, housing, diet, transport, employment and self-esteem.

New patterns of exclusion in health have included the following: (i) the establishment of a two-tier structure of access to health services through the system of GP fundholding, which accompanied the introduction of the 'internal market' in the NHS (Pollock 1997, Le Grand *et al.* 1998), together with the active encouragement by government of the expansion of the UK private health care sector since 1979 (Harrison *et al.* 1990, Ham 1992); (ii) the increase in homelessness generated by New Right policies, with a consequent expansion in the numbers of individuals and families living in circumstances that endanger their health (Davies 1993), who experience difficulty in accessing health care (The Big Issue in the North Trust 1998), and whose needs continue to be both ignored by the NHS structure and stereotyped in the hostile images of 'able-bodied beggars' or 'too smelly, too dirty and often too drunk' down-and-outs with which many health professionals operate (Fisher and Collins 1993); and (iii) the inability of those with the poorest health to engage with governments' health promotion strategies, which call for us all to take responsibility for our health, make the healthy choice and change our lifestyles accordingly (DOH 1992, 1998).

In this collection two further chapters examine effects in the health field of Thatcherite New Right ideology and the increase in exclusion that has followed in its wake.

Blackburn (Chapter 2) focuses on the experiences of low-income households with children and offers a clear account of the nature and extent of this vulnerable group's exclusion from good health. Exclusion from good health is shown to be a significant dimension of poverty and to be affected by 'social and health policy and practice'. The chapter examines three dimensions of health exclusion, discussing how low-income families are excluded from 'membership of a "healthy" society', from 'healthy lifestyles' and from 'responsive health care provision'. Blackburn emphasises the ways in which the attitudes of health professionals to poverty and to the poor can contribute to reducing their access to appropriate health care and concludes by discussing the role of health practitioners in tackling health exclusion, a role which involves incorporating a poverty perspective in their work.

Purdy (Chapter 4) addresses the exclusion of those with the poorest health from the 'healthy lifestyles' promoted by the Tory government, and more recently by New Labour's health promotion strategy for England. Both *The Health of the Nation* (DOH 1992) and *Our Healthier Nation* (DOH 1998) share in a view of health which suggests that preventable illness and premature death can largely be avoided if individuals and families are more careful about the lifestyles they choose. Purdy suggests that this focus on individual responsibility for health and on 'making the healthy choice' reinforces an inverse care law that perpetuates inequalities in health. The structural contexts in which choices and compromises are made are largely ignored, and 'unhealthy' lifestyles and behaviours are easily dismissed as irresponsible and socially deviant.

The link between health promotion and social regulation is discussed, with health promotion discourses functioning to encourage and endorse 'specific attitudes towards health and associated practices of "self regulation" '. Purdy argues that in the emerging new consensus on welfare, policing of the healthy self is pivotal to citizenship, with the 'duty to be healthy' marking out a significant dimension for the social construction of the responsible citizen, family and community. As such, the 'healthism' present in health strategies such as *The Health of the Nation* and *Our Healthier Nation* risks excluding and demonising different and minority lifestyles which do not fit cleanly into the 'healthy norm'.

Exclusion in health work

The discourse of New Right ideology has also impacted on exclusion in health work, through the deregulation of the health market, with the establishing of a policy of contracting-out for ancillary and support services in the NHS (Rivett 1998), and through the dominance of 'managerialism' and 'consumerism', which present significant challenges to professional authority in health matters.

It is important to note, however, that New Right discourses of managerialism and consumerism are not the only challenges to professional, and especially medical, dominance and authority in the field of health. Other significant challenges to medical hegemony lie in the questioning of the effectiveness of medical interventions in enhancing health mounted, for example, by the World Health Organisation (WHO 1978, 1984, 1986a, 1998). Here the call is for an 'intersectoral' approach to health promotion in which health is viewed as the responsibility of agencies other than medicine and in which community involvement and empowerment are key processes and aims (WHO 1978, 1981, 1985, 1986b, 1988). Medicine is also under challenge from the rise of 'user' groups who question the right of health professionals to determine the health agenda and the services offered (see for example, Kelleher 1994, Stacey 1994, Morris 1995, Barnes 1997, Croft and Beresford 1998). Finally, Freidson's pessimistic assessment of medical power remaining effectively unchallenged (Freidson 1970, 1994) may need to be reviewed in the wake of public disquiet over high-profile events that question medical competence, such as the recent Bristol cardiothoracic 'scandal', and that prompt promises of government action to increase the public accountability of both individual medical practitioners and the profession itself.

Conflict over professional authority in health is not, then, simply reducible to the impact of New Right ideology. Indeed, it would appear that support for certain shifts in power within health professions is to be found in both Tory and New Labour policies. The ascendancy of GPs *vis-à-vis* hospital consultants, for example, is aided by *both* the establishment of GP fundholding (DOH 1989) and the current government's plans to abolish fundholding in favour of 'primary care groups' (DOH 1997). For both initiatives signal government's intention of creating a primary-care-led NHS. They also suggest that a shift in the balance of power within medicine may be occurring, challenging the post-war experience, which has seen the marginalisation of both public health medicine and general practice in relation to the 'medical dominance' exercised by hospital-based consultants in the acute sector (Bury 1997). Such shifts in the balance of power within medicine testify to the existence of internal divisions within the medical and allied health professions and to the fact that 'these divisions may be intensifying in response to health service reforms' (Annandale 1998: 248).

In directing attention to exclusion in health work it is important to recognise two dimensions. First, exclusion exists in the form of barriers to participation in health work. Here certain individuals, groups and some professions experience limits to their practice which reflect the degree of authority they possess or lack in the health field.

Two chapters in the present volume examine aspects of exclusion in health work which focus on this operation of power and authority. In the first, the need to reject any notion of exclusion as a simple binary process is demonstrated by Fox (Chapter 7) in an analysis of a set of interactions between doctors and patients in negotiating discharge from hospital following surgery. Whilst the 'doctor–patient' relationship has long been a central focus of medical sociology (Bury 1997), what distinguishes Fox's analysis is the post-structuralist and postmodern approach (Fox 1993) employed to examine the ways in which doctors are able to achieve authority over patients and thereby effectively exclude their 'voices' from the decision-making process regarding discharge. Utilising concepts drawn from post-structuralism. Fox develops a 'deconstructive strategy' with which to look at the negotiations between doctors and patients. This approach reveals new dimensions to the interactions between health professionals and patients, interactions which 'usually' but not inevitably sustain 'medical definitions of situations'.

Although 'deconstruction' enables us to see how medical discourse is able to establish its authority, by identifying the strategies through which a medical reading of the situation becomes privileged over alternative readings, its value really lies in its ability to overturn privileged readings and thereby offer a basis for resistance and, in this case, a challenge to medical hegemony. The significance of a post-structuralist approach is to confirm that authority – that is, 'the capacity to be acknowledged as "speaking the truth" ' – is never fixed or settled but is constantly subject to resistance. Thus the ability of medicine to dominate the health field requires it to reaffirm itself and win the struggle for power in its daily practices. Fox concludes that 'deconstruction' is not merely a methodology for qualitative data analysis but also 'a political tool which opposes authoritarian exercises of power'. As such, a post-structuralist and postmodern approach offers a valuable perspective with which to consider how practices of exclusion are achieved and sustained, and how they might be better challenged.

The power and authority of medical discourse and its role in promoting and sustaining exclusion in health is also identified by Kirkham (Chapter 5) in a historical account of the development of exclusion in maternity care. This illustrates the process by which male medical and professional control and management of an arena of health care has been achieved with exclusionary repercussions, in this case for both midwives and mothers.

From a pre-industrial situation in which birth existed as 'the pivot of a female culture', Kirkham documents the impact of processes of professionalisation and the institutionalisation of health care on what had previously been 'women's business'. In this process, the definition of the 'right way to give birth' shifted from women themselves to medicine and therefore to men. Women and the midwives who attended them became excluded from decision-making, and birth became constructed in terms of a male, medical discourse.

The impact of the 'imperative of professionalisation' on midwifery saw the power associated with professional status being restricted to particular groups of midwives, a development which effectively excluded working-class midwives. Kirkham emphasises the professionalisation of midwifery required a shift of allegiance from patient to doctor. Midwives increasingly internalised the values of medicine, which today structure both their training and their practice. In short, 'obstetrics has colonised normal birth', and the requirement of expert knowledge and status has 'fundamentally changed midwives' relationships with childbearing women'.

Kirkham shows how a double exclusion operates in the arena of maternity care: the exclusion of female health professionals by the authority of (male) medical interventions, and of female labouring by female health professionals. One significant effect of the latter is for an inverse care law to operate in midwifery practice, according to which, for example, the information labouring women receive from midwives may be more closely linked to their social class than to their needs. The chapter concludes with a discussion of the possibilities of challenging exclusion in maternity care and of re-establishing partnerships between midwives and childbearing women.

Kirkham's analysis of the exclusion of female labouring by mid-wives points to a second dimension of exclusion in health work in which health professionals 'collaborate', intentionally or otherwise, in producing and reproducing relations of exclusion through their practice in a variety of ways. This second dimension emphasises the 'policing', 'surveillance' and 'regulatory' activity performed by health professionals, a focus developed, for example, in 'social construction-ist' accounts of the 'surveillance' function of health promotion and public health discourses (see for example, Bunton 1992, Bunton and Burrows 1995, Lupton 1995, Nettleton and Bunton 1995, Nettleton 1997, and Purdy Chapter 4 of this volume).

In this collection Morrall (Chapter 6) examines the 'collaboration' of psychiatric medicine and mental health nursing in 'the governance of the mentally disordered on behalf of the state'. Historically, the 'powerful' have segregated and marginalised the 'insane'. In the nineteenth century this found expression in the building of asylums into which the 'mad' and the unreasonable could be physically segregated from society. Significantly this 'first psychiatric revolution' enabled medicine and nursing to establish their right to survey the madness. By the end of the century medicine had secured its 'monopolisation of the care of the mentally ill'.

Morrall argues that, despite the contemporary move away from the asylum as the site for psychiatric and nursing care, the surveil-lance and policing of the 'mad' continues to be undertaken by health professionals in other locations. Psychiatric medicine and mental health nursing have extended their social control functions out of the asylum and into the community, and Morrall rejects any notion that the relocation of the 'mentally disordered' into the community has fragmented or challenged their control by health professionals. Indeed, current government policy is shown to favour the 'recarceration' of the mentally ill in the community and to call for the psychiatric professions to increase rather than decrease their regulation of the 'mad'.

Exclusion operates at a number of different levels and in many different sites in the field of health care and health work. Conse-quently, a problem in explaining its presence and its persistence involves the question of how to make sense of its complex configura-tion without simply reducing its many facets to the outcome of some central site or fundamental source of origin for all exclusionary policies and practices. Thus, for example, the attraction of simply laying the responsibility for exclusion in health during the 1980s and 1990s at the door of New Right ideology must be resisted, insofar as it (i) denies the significance of patterns of exclusion in health which were already established before 1979, (ii) ignores the significance of other forces in promoting such inequalities, (iii) assumes that the process of implementing central government policy actually works, and (iv) implies that exclusion might be removed by a change in political ideology. All of these notions require careful examination if the phenomena of exclusion in health are to be addressed and fought.

Exclusion under New Labour

Just as continuities and discontinuities in the pattern of exclusion in health care and in health work can be identified during the last fifty years, so the form that exclusion will take following the election of a New Labour government can be expected to display both links and breaks with the past. The forms of exclusion in health which we can expect will very much depend on the terms of any new consensus on welfare which the present government and others achieve. Already this new (post-Fordist) consensus over welfare may be beginning to take shape, indicated by the elements of Tory New Right thinking which Labour now appears to endorse and even seems to want to extend further. These elements are those associated with the neo-conservative wing of Thatcherism, namely a concern for re-establishing moral authority and social duty expressed through the central role reserved for the 'family' as the key site for securing social integration and mutual cooperation.

Labour's 'third way' promises to maintain continuity with neo-conservativism whilst distancing itself from the excesses of neo-liberal individualism. The unrestrained competition of the free market is to be curbed, but then so are opportunities for state welfarism. On balance, third way thinking handles the market 'gently' (Hunter 1998). There is to be no return to collectivism. Instead, New Labour is committed to 'communitarianism' (Etzioni 1993), in which both state and market are rejected in favour of 'community' (Clarke 1996). For New Labour, the 'responsible family' is to be the foundation upon which communities can be built and society moved forward (Home Office 1998). In this communitarian vision 'Social justice is reworked as community and individual obligation' (Hughes and Mooney 1998: 98).

So what effect is New Labour's third way likely to have on health and exclusion? Whilst we may reasonably hope that the government will not champion consumerism in the NHS and thereby support the increasing exclusion of those sections of the population poorly placed to act as consumers, its refusal to rediscover and reinvest in ideals of social justice and the necessity for state welfarism signals a potentially dangerous future for the NHS. For New Labour's rejection of both 'command and control' and 'free market' models of health care in its plans for a new NHS (DOH 1997, Baker 1998) invites the possibility of primary care groups excluding high-risk and vulnerable groups from their purchasing plans as they take on the commissioning of services for large populations together with the responsibility for local rationing of these services in order to stay within their 'capped' budgets. New Labour's third way risks extending the experience of exclusion in health and health care, and in its creation of primary care groups 'disposing of the central tenets of equity and universal coverage and NHS care free at the point of delivery' (Pollock 1998: 28).

Only by re-embracing collectivist ideals can New Labour achieve an NHS committed to reducing exclusion and inequalities in health and health care. The third way cannot deliver this.

Challenging exclusion

To emphasise that exclusion in health is not a recent phenomenon but one that pre-dates both the New Right ideology of Thatcherism and the communitarianism of New Labour is not to conclude that the marginalisation of sections of the British population from the experiences of health and well-being enjoyed by the rest of us is either inevitable or acceptable. Many of the contributors to this volume draw attention to the issue of challenging exclusion in health and, despite differences in perspective, all recognise the existence of exclusionary practices in the field of health and the need to engage critically with these practices.

The relations of power, control and regulation that underpin exclusion and inequality in health are never complete. The implementation of exclusionary policies and strategies is never totally predictable and may be contradictory or give rise to unanticipated effects. Consumerism, for example, may provide opportunities for individual empowerment as services are forced to 'get closer to the customer', although this does beg the question as to the conditions under which health service users and workers can effectively exert their influence and secure their choices. For the possibility of challenging exclusion in health involves more than encouraging individuals to become better consumers and make better and more informed choices. It also involves action by health professionals and by government.

Action by health professionals involves recognising the political nature of their work. This may be uncomfortable, insofar as professionalisation presents itself as a politically neutral process. In addition, contemporary nursing practice favours a focus on individualised patient care which can prevent nurses from developing a population approach and public health orientation in their work (Purdy 1997). In the field of health promotion this has contributed to nursing's general acceptance of a 'narrow lifestyle orientated definition of health promotion' and a tendency to ignore the impact of structural inequalities on individuals' health-related behaviour (Brown and Piper 1997). The need for nurses to recognise the political nature of their work and apply a sociological perspective is crucial, given New Labour's aproach to public health, which continues rather than rejects the Tory tendency to 'blame the victim' (Purdy 1998).

Blackburn (1996) describes some of the ways in which health visitors have attempted to move away from 'individualistic forms of practice' in responding to the scale of health inequalities and poverty which they encounter in Britain today. This has involved the development of 'proactive health visiting', in which a teamwork approach to practice is central. In this volume, Blackburn (Chapter 2) again calls for health visitors to develop a poverty perspective in their practice in order that they might better challenge policies that promote health exclusion and assist families to deal with the effects of poverty on health. This requires that health professionals' negative attitudes towards poverty and those on low income are effectively challenged in order that ways of working can be developed which confirm to families 'that they are not to blame for their poor health'.

The need for health professionals to forge new relationships with their clients if exclusion in health is to be challenged is taken up by Kirkham (Chapter 5), who argues that the development of a 'partnership' between midwives and childbearing women may be effective in challenging the exclusion experienced by both. Such partnerships between health professional and 'service user' signify both the empowerment of the client and the willingness of health professionals to give up a degree of power and authority associated with their traditional relationships with patients. However difficult moves towards 'power sharing' in the health field may be, it is clear that they are central to any serious attempt to challenge exclusion. In short, challenging exclusion in health requires that the individuals, groups and communities who experience exclusion are empowered by the actions of the health professionals working alongside them.

Whilst empowerment may be decisive in challenging exclusion in health, it cannot be assumed to be a simple or straightforward process. Walker (Chapter 9), for example, suggests that an important issue for health care systems is just how to 'promote the *participation* of older people and their family carers' in processes from which they have traditionally been excluded. For here is a group of service users and their carers who have previously been encouraged to remain silent and dependent by the exercise of professional power. Their participation requires, amongst other things, that services be more open to user involvement, with bureaucratic provider-led models of service organisation being replaced by more responsive needs-led and user-orientated systems. In identifying a number of 'key principles of empowerment' to assist health and social care workers develop more empowering approaches, Walker emphasises that empowerment is not about increasing competition between individuals. Rather, it is, or should be, 'a collective as well as an individual process'.

Recognising the social and collective nature of the empowerment process is central to challenging exclusion in health, insofar as it points to the importance of health professionals exploring the possibilities of a 'community approach' to issues of exclusion and inequalities in health. Identifying the role of 'structural' features, such as unemployment, poverty and poor housing, in generating health inequalities and poor and unequal access to health care resources supports a 'commnuity development' approach to health promotion, an approach which seeks to protect and improve health by empowering communities. In the present volume, Davies (Chapter 8) offers an example of this approach, discussing and detailing the evaluation of a recent project in East London which highlights both the benefits and challenges of the approach.

The overall benefit of a community development approach lies in the fact that, as Davies states, 'empowering communities to identify their own health needs and facilitating ways to address those needs can be a health enhancing activity'. But the approach also raises a number of difficult issues. These include the problem of ensuring that the agenda is set by the community itself rather than by health professionals, and the difficulties associated with encouraging all voices in the community to be heard rather than only those of a vocal minority. In the context of the East London project on which Davies is reporting, difficulties are noted in both generating community involvement in the first place and in maintaining this involvement. Furthermore, the potential for community concerns to be marginalised in the face of the requirement for health professionals to 'achieve government imposed targets in relation to specific health indicators' is noted.

Although health professionals, in partnership with others, clearly can have an impact on exclusion in health, it is essential to acknowledge the limits of this action. An emphasis on 'community', for example, can suggest that health problems, including exclusion from health resources and barriers to accessing both primary and secondary health services, are resolvable at a community level. According to this scenario, all that is necessary is greater effort and cooperation between health and social care professionals, local authorities and other agencies and communities themselves for exclusion and inequalities in health to be effectively reduced. New Labour's 'third way' endorses this thinking with its emphasis on local 'partnerships', 'healthy living centres' and 'health action zones'. Unfortunately, just as 'decentralisation' may contain the promise of greater local community control, it can 'also be used to justify central government's abdication from particular areas of responsibility' (Mayo 1994: 15). In the case of New Labour, a striking example of this tendency is its continuance of the Tory government's strategy of delegating responsibility for identifying, tackling and reducing inequalities, or as the previous government preferred to call them, 'variations' in health, to local initiatives.

Whilst the delegation of responsibility for the 'nation's health' to the nation itself may sit comfortably with both New Right and New Labour ideologies, the tendency shared by both of reducing the role of the state in providing adequate welfare resources cannot be justified in the face of the exclusion and inequalities in health to which the contributors to this volume and others elsewhere draw attention. Only central government action can affect the 'structural' changes necessary if the forces and conditions which encourage exclusion in health are to be significantly challenged. The structural changes required have been well documented, and demand a 'strategy of redistribution' (Townsend 1997). They include central government action on income, unemployment and housing (Benzeval *et al.* 1995, Acheson 1998). Refusal to consider such central government action will only reinforce New Labour's current tendency to restrict its public health strategy to a narrow, medically-dominated approach (Peckham *et al.* 1998). If New Labour is serious about prioritising public health, then it must change its approach to challenging social exclusion and poverty. The form and direction of the welfare restructuring which the 'global economic order' appears to require of it is not predetermined or inevitable. The third way cannot be allowed to be the only way.

References

Acheson, D. (chair) (1998) *Independent Inquiry into Inequalities in Health Report*, London: The Stationery Office.

Alcock, P. (1996) *Social Policy in Britain: Themes and Issues*, London: Macmillan.

Allen, J. (1992) 'Post-industrialism and post-Fordism', in S. Hall, D. Held and T. McGrew (eds) *Modernity and its Futures*, Cambridge: Polity Press/The Open University.

Allsop, J. (1995) 'Health: from seamless service to patchwork quilt', in D. Gladstone (ed.) *British Social Welfare: Past, Present and Future*, London: UCL Press.

Amin, A. (1994) 'Post-Fordism: models, fantasies and phantoms of transition', in A. Amin (ed.) *Post-Fordism: A Reader*, Oxford: Blackwell.

Annandale, E. (1998) *The Sociology of Health and Medicine: A Critical Introduction*, Cambridge: Polity Press.

Baggott, B. (1994) *Health and Health Care in Britain*, London: Macmillan.

Baker, M. (1998) *Making Sense of the NHS White Paper*, Abingdon: Radcliffe Medical Press.

Baldock, J. and Ungerson, C. (1996) 'Becoming a consumer of care: developing a sociological account of the "new community care" ', in S. Edgell, K. Hetherington and A. Warde (eds) *Consumption Matters: The Production and Experience of Consumption*, Oxford: Blackwell Publishers/The Sociological Review.

Baldwin, S. and Falkingham, J. (eds) (1994) *Social Security and Social Change: New Challenges to the Beveridge Model*, London: Harvester Wheatsheaf.

Barnes, M. (1997) *Care, Communities and Citizens*, London: Longman.

Benzeval, M. (1997) 'Health', in A. Walker and C. Walker (eds) *Britain Divided: The Growth of Social Exclusion in the 1980s and 1990s*, London: CAPG.

Benzeval, M., Judge, K. and Whitehead, M. (eds) (1995) *Tackling Inequalities in Health: An Agenda for Action*, London: King's Fund.

Berridge, V. and Webster, C. (1993) 'The crisis of welfare, 1974 to the 1980s', in C. Webster (ed.) *Caring For Health: History and Diversity*, revised edition, Ballmore: Open University Press.

Blackburn, C. (1996) 'Building a poverty perspective into health visiting practice', in P. Bywaters and E. McLeod (eds) *Working for Equality in Health*, London: Routledge.

Brown, P.A. and Piper, S.M. (1997) 'Nursing and the health of the nation: schism or symbiosis?', *Journal of Advanced Nursing* 25, 297–301.

Bunton, R. (1992) 'More than a woolly jumper: health promotion as social regulation', *Critical Public Health* 3, 2: 4–11.

Bunton, R. and Burrows, R. (1995) 'Consumption and health in the "epidemiological" clinic of late modern medicine', in R. Bunton, S. Nettleton and R. Burrows (eds) *The Sociology of Health Promotion: Critical Analyses of Consumption, Lifestyle and Risk*, London: Routledge.

Burrows, R. and Loader, B. (eds) (1994) *Towards a Post-Fordist Welfare State?*, London: Routledge.

Bury, M. (1997) *Health and Illness in a Changing Society*, London: Routledge.

Butler, J. (1992) *Patients, Policies and Politics: Before and After Working For Patients*, Buckingham: Open University Press.

Carter, J. (ed.) (1998) *Postmodernity and the Fragmentation of Welfare*, London: Routledge.

Clarke, J. (1996) 'Public nightmares and communitarian dreams: the crisis of the social in social welfare', in S. Edgell, K. Hetherington and A. Wardle (eds) *Consumption Matters: The Production and Experience of Consumption*, Oxford: Blackwell Publishers/The Sociological Review.

Clarke, J. and Newman, J. (1997) *The Managerial State: Power, Politics and Ideology in the Remaking of Social Welfare*, London: Sage.

Cochrane, A. (1993) 'Comparative approaches and social policy', in A. Cochrane and J. Clarke (eds) *Comparing Welfare States: Britain in International Context*, London: Sage/The Open University.

Croft, S. and Beresford, P. (1998) 'Postmodernity and the future of welfare: whose critiques, whose social policy?', in J. Carter (ed.) *Postmodernity and the Fragmentation of Welfare*, London: Routledge.

Davies, E. (1993) 'The health of the homeless', in A. Beattie, M. Gott, L. Jones and M. Sidell (eds) *Health and Wellbeing: A Reader*, London: Macmillan/The Open University.

Deacon, B. (with Hulse, M. and Stubbs, P.) (1997) *Global Social Policy: International Organizations and the Future of Welfare*, London: Sage.

Department of Health (DOH) (1989) *Working For Patients*, London: HMSO.

——(1992) *The Health of the Nation: A Strategy for Health in England*, London: HMSO.

——(1995) *The Health of the Nation: Variations in Health. What Can the Department of Health and the NHS Do?*, Report of the Variations Sub-Group of the Chief Medical Officer's Health of the Nation Working Group, London: DOH.

——(1997) *The New NHS: Modern, Dependable*, London: The Stationery Office.

——(1998) *Our Healthier Nation: A Contract for Health*, London: The Stationery Office.

Drever, F. and Whitehead, M. (eds) (1997) *Health Inequalities*, Office for National Statistics, London: The Stationery Office.

Edgell, S. and Hetherington, K. (1996) 'Introduction: consumption matters', in S. Edgell, K. Hetherington and A. Wardle (eds) *Consumption Matters: The Production and Experience of Consumption*, Oxford: Blackwell Publishers/The Sociological Review.

Etzioni, A. (1993) *The Spirit of Community: Rights, Responsibilities and the Communitarian Agenda*, London: Fontana Press.

Fisher, K. and Collins, J. (eds) (1993) *Homelessness, Health Care and Welfare Provision*, London: Routledge.

Fox, N.J. (1993) *Postmodernism, Sociology and Health*, Buckingham: Open University Press.

Freidson, E. (1970) *Profession of Medicine: A Study of the Sociology of Applied Knowledge*, London: University of Chicago Press.

——(1994) *Professionalism Reborn: Theory, Prophecy and Policy*, Cambridge: Polity Press.

Gamble, A. (1994) *The Free Economy and the Strong State: The Politics of Thatcherism*, second edition, London: Macmillan.

Glennerster, H. (1990) 'Social policy since the Second World War', in J. Hills (ed.) *The State of Welfare: The Welfare State in Britain since 1974*, Oxford: Clarendon Press.

Ham, C. (1992) *Health Policy in Britain: The Politics and Organisation of the National Health Service*, third edition, London: Macmillan.

Harrison, S., Hunter, D.J. and Pollitt, C. (1990) *The Dynamics of British Health Policy*, London: Routledge.

Hindess, B. (1987) *Freedom, Equality and the Market: Arguments on Social Policy*, London: Tavistock.

Home Office (1998) *Supporting Families: A Consultation Document*, London: The Stationery Office.

Hughes, G. and Mooney, G. (1998) 'Community', in G. Hughes (ed.) *Imagining Welfare Futures*, London: Routledge/The Open University.

Hunter, D. (1998) 'Which way lies the third way?', *Health Service Journal* 108, 5615: 16–17.

Johnson, N. (1990) *Reconstructing the Welfare State: A Decade of Change 1980–1990*, London: Harvester Wheatsheaf.

Kelleher, D. (1994) 'Self-help groups and their relationship to medicine', in J. Gabe, D. Kelleher and G. Williams (eds) *Challenging Medicine*, London: Routledge.

Kendall, I. and Moon, G. (1994) 'Health policy and the Conservatives', in S. Savage, R. Atkinson and L. Robins (eds) *Public Policy in Britain*, London: St Martin's Press.

Klein, R. (1995) *The New Politics of the National Health Service*, third edition, London: Longman.

Le Grand, J. (1982) *The Strategy of Equality*, London: George Allen and Unwin.

Le Grand, J., Mays, N. and Mulligan, J. (eds) (1998) *Learning from the NHS Internal Market*, London: King's Fund.

Lupton, D. (1995) *The Imperative of Health: Public Health and the Regulated Body*, London: Sage.

Mayer, M. (1994) 'Post-Fordist city politics', in A. Amin (ed.) *Post-Fordism: A Reader*, Oxford: Blackwell.

Mayo, M. (1994) *Communities and Caring: The Mixed Economy of Welfare*, London: St Martin's Press.

Morris, J. (1995) 'Creating a space for absent voices: disabled women's experience of receiving assistance with daily living activities', in M. Allott and M. Robb (eds) *Understanding Health and Social Care: An Introductory Reader*, London: Sage/The Open University.

Nettleton, S. (1997) 'Surveillance, health promotion and the formation of a risk identity', in M. Sidell, L. Jones, J. Katz and A. Peberdy (eds) *Debates and Dilemmas in Promoting Health: A Reader*, London: Macmillan/The Open University.

Nettleton, S. and Bunton, R. (1995) 'Sociological critiques of health promotion', in R. Bunton, S. Nettleton and R. Burrows (eds) *The Sociology of Health Promotion: Critical Analyses of Consumption, Lifestyle and Risk*, London: Routledge.

O'Brien, M. and Penna, S. (1998) *Theorising Welfare: Enlightenment and Modern Society*, London: Sage.

Peckham, S., Taylor, P. and Turton, P. (1998) 'An unhealthy focus on illness', *Health Matters* 33, Spring 1998, 8–10.

Phillimore, P., Beattie, A. and Townsend, P. (1994) 'Widening inequality of health in northern England, 1981–91', *British Medical Journal* 308: 1125–8.

Pollock, A. (1997) 'Rationing in the "reformed" NHS', in S. Iliffe and J. Munro (eds) *Healthy Choices: Future Options for the NHS*, London: Lawrence and Wishart.

——(1998) 'The American way', *Health Service Journal* 108, 5599: 28–9.

Purdy, M. (1997) 'Is nursing anti-social?', *Nursing Times* 92, 20: 42–4.

——(1998) 'Sick...and tired of stereotypes', *Nursing Standard* 13, 4: 26–7.

Ranade, W. (1994) *A Future for the NHS? Health Care in the 1990s*, London: Longman.

Rhodes, R.A.W. (1997) *Understanding Governance: Policy Networks, Governance, Reflexivity and Accountability*, Buckingham: Open University Press.

Richardson, A. and Reid, G. (1997) *Sheffield and Electoral Ward Mortality Trends, 1981 to 1996*, Sheffield: Sheffield Health, Department of Information and Research.

Rivett, G. (1998) *From Cradle to Grave: Fifty Years of the NHS*, London: King's Fund.

Shaw, M., Dorling, D. and Brimblecombe, N (1998) 'Changing the map: health in Britain, 1951–1991', *Sociology of Health and Medicine* 20, 5: 694–709.

Stacey, M. (1994) 'The power of lay knowledge: a personal view', in J. Popay and G. Williams (eds) *Researching the People's Health*, London: Routledge.

The Big Issue in the North Trust (1998) *A Primary Care Study of Vendors of The Big Issue in the North*, Manchester: The Big Issue in the North Trust.

Townsend, P. (1997) 'Redistribution: the strategic alternative to privatisation', in A. Walker and C. Walker (eds) *Britain Divided: The Growth of Social Exclusion in the 1980s and 1990s*, London: CPAG.

Townsend, P. and Davidson, N. (eds) (1982) *The Black Report*, in P. Townsend, M. Whitehead and N. Davidson (eds) *Inequalities in Health: The Black Report and the Health Divide*, London: Penguin Books.

Walker, A. (1993) 'Community care policy: from consensus to conflict', in J. Bornat, C. Pereira, D. Pilgrim and F. Williams (eds) *Community Care: A Reader*, London: Macmillan/The Open University.

——(1997) 'Community care: past, present and future', in S. Iliffe and J. Munro (eds) *Healthy Choices: Future Options for the NHS*, London: Lawrence and Wishart.

Walker, A. and Walker, C. (1997) 'Conclusion: prioritise poverty now', in A. Walker and C. Walker (eds) *Britain Divided: The Growth of Social Exclusion in the 1980s and 1990s*, London: CAPG.

Whitehead, M (1992) *The Health Divide*, in P. Townsend, M. Whitehead and N. Davidson (eds) *Inequalities in Health: The Black Report and the Health Divide*, London Penguin Books.

Williams, F. (1993) 'Gender, "race" and class in British welfare policy', in A. Cochrane and J. Clarke (eds) *Comparing Welfare States: Britain in International Context*, London: Sage/The Open University.

World Health Organisation (WHO) (1978) *Report on the International Conference on Primary Health Care*, Alma Ata, 6–12 September, Geneva: WHO.

——(1981) *Regional Strategy for Attaining Health for All by the Year 2000*, Copenhagen: WHO.

——(1984) *Health Promotion: A Discussion Document on the Concept and Principles*, Copenhagen: WHO.

——(1985) *Targets for Health For All: Targets in Support of the Regional Strategy for Health For All*, Copenhagen: WHO Regional Office for Europe.

——(1986a) *Intersectoral Action for Health: The Role of Intersectoral Co-operation in National Strategies for Health for All*, Geneva: WHO.

——(1986b) *The Ottowa Charter for Health Promotion*, Copenhagen: WHO.

——(1988) *Promoting Health in the Urban Context*, WHO Healthy Cities Project, Paper No. 1, Copenhagen: FADL.

——(1998) *Health 21: The Health for All Policy for the WHO European Region: 21 Targets for the 21st Century*, Copenhagen: WHO Regional Office for Europe.

2 Poor health, poor health care

The experiences of low-income households with children

Clare Blackburn

Introduction

This chapter focuses on the experiences of low-income households with children, documenting the extent and nature of their exclusion from good health. Adults and children in poverty have more illnesses, more disabilities and shorter lives that their better-off counterparts. As a group, not only are their health care needs greater than those of more affluent groups, they are also different. Reducing poverty is key to improving the health of low-income groups and tackling social inequalities in health. However, the evidence suggests that poverty levels have risen and social inequalities in health have widened. Over the last decade, a strong theme developed in the literature on poverty has been the link between the poverty and social exclusion. Writers have documented the development of new social divisions and the interrelated forms of social exclusion that have emerged (Lister 1990, 1997, Room 1995, Walker 1997). While many of these discussions focus on the notions of poverty, citizenship and social exclusion, they draw attention, although often only in an oblique fashion, to health exclusion as a dimension of poverty. As social divisions and poverty are corrosive of full citizenship (Lister 1997), they are also corrosive of full health.

This chapter draws attention to the way social and health policy and practice exclude low-income households from good health and responsive health care provision. It begins with a brief discussion of the scale and distribution of poverty in Britain today. This provides the backdrop to, and a way of contextualising, health exclusion in poverty. The chapter then moves on to examine three dimensions of health exclusion, drawing attention to the way low-income households with children are victims of exclusionary health and social policies and practices. First, it discusses how low-income families are excluded from membership of a 'healthy' society. Through a brief discussion of inequalities in health and the widening health gap between poor and better-off families, it documents how low-income households with children have shorter lives, more illnesses and disabilities and greater stress and distress than their better-off counterparts. Second, and as a way of partially explaining the first dimension of health exclusion, it explores how low-income families are excluded from healthy lifestyles. Drawing on evidence from studies on housing conditions, eating patterns and cigarette smoking behaviour, it illustrates how access to vital health resources is reduced and health behaviour is constrained when money is short and health care burdens are heavy. The third dimension of health exclusion documented in this chapter is low-income households' exclusion from responsive health care provision. In doing so, it draws attention not only to the barriers to access but also to the way that health care practitioner attitudes to poverty and poor clients, and their failure to incorporate a poverty perspective in their work, combine to reduce the access of adults and children in poverty to appropriate health care. Finally, the chapter discusses the role of health practitioners in tackling health exclusion. It limits its discussion, primarily to households with dependent children, and seeks to provide an illustrative rather than comprehensive discussion of the nature and extent of health exclusion in poverty.

Today's poverty

There is nothing new about poverty, nor is it unique to Britain. Although it was not uncommon in the 1980s and early 1990s to hear government ministers proclaim that poverty no longer existed, it is now generally accepted that poverty, both absolute and relative, continues to be a major social issue which is undermining the social and economic fabric of British society. Several things are notable about today's poverty. First, the scale of poverty in Britain; second, the distribution of poverty between different groups; and third, the deterioration in the material position of families in poverty.

Poverty levels have been on the increase since the late 1970s. Regardless of the poverty indicator selected, the figures suggest that there has been a substantial increase in the number and proportions of individuals and households in poverty in the 1990s. Using the commonly adopted poverty line of below 50 per cent of average income (which is made available through a set of government statistics called *Households Below Average Income Statistics*), the proportion of people living in poverty increased from 9 per cent of the population (5 million people) in 1979 to 24 per cent of the population (nearly 14 million people) in 1993/4 (DSS 1996). These figures, while providing valuable information about the scale of poverty in the population as a whole, hide the distribution of poverty between different social groups. Households with children are the largest single group in poverty. This can be explained largely by the fact that the two major causes of poverty over the last two decades, unemployment and low pay, have had a disproportionate effect on households with children. In 1993/4, 28 per cent of households with children had incomes below 50 per cent of average income after housing costs (DSS 1996). As a result, a third (32 per cent) of children in Britain live in poverty. This compares to 10 per cent of children in 1979. As a result of growing poverty levels, a significant number of households with young children are dependent on income support, the key safety-net social security benefit. Between 1979 and 1996 there has been a three-fold increase in households with children in receipt of income support, from 0.5 million to 1.5 million (DSS 1980, 1997). Although there have been some changes in the distribution of poverty among different types of households, one thing remains unchanged: the disproportionate shouldering of the poverty burden by Black and minority ethnic groups, women (particularly lone mothers), and disabled people.

A third feature of today's poverty is that the increase in the proportions of people in poverty has been accompanied by a deterioration in the financial circumstances of the poor. Walker suggests that there is evidence of 'desperate poverty on a scale not witnessed in Britain since the 1930s' (Walker 1997). The *Households Below Average Income Statistics* documents rising income inequalities over the 1980s and early 1990s. While average real incomes increased by 40 per cent, after housing costs, between 1979 and 1993/4, the real incomes of the poorest 10 per cent of the population decreased by 13 per cent, after housing costs (DSS 1996). Goodman and Webb's analysis of the changing distribution of income in the UK (1994) also suggests that the real incomes of the poorest tenth of the population, after housing costs, fell sharply between 1961 and 1991, representing a return to the living standards of the mid-1960s.

It is widely accepted that poverty is multi-dimensional and that low income has a range of consequences and dimensions for individuals and society as a whole. In the discussion that follows, this chapter draws attention to the way that low income shapes people's health quality and health experience, excluding them from good health, healthy lifestyles and health service provision.

Excluded from good health

Across a range of health measures, there is strong evidence that poor people are excluded from good health. Those who live in the poorest financial, social and material circumstances have shorter lives, experience more illnesses and disability and greater distress than their better-off counterparts. A number of studies document how people in low-income groups are excluded from long, healthy lives. The most widely used indicator of social and economic position is social class. Although it does not directly reflect financial position, it reflects inequalities in power, status and access to resources. Social class measures are commonly used to distinguish variations in mortality and morbidity between groups. The *Longitudinal Study* provides detailed data on adult mortality by social class and other socio-economic indicators, such as car ownership and housing tenure. For both men and women, death rates are highest in the lowest social class and lowest in the highest social class (Goldblatt 1990). A similar pattern emerges if asset-based indicators, which are thought to be more effective discriminators of health status than social class, are used: men and women in more advantaged circumstances have lower death rates than those in disadvantaged circumstances (ibid.). Infant and child mortality rates also show a sharp gradient by social class at all ages but not for all causes of death (Woodroffe *et al.* 1993). However, there is not a main cause of death for which children in lower social classes have relatively lower rates than children in higher social classes.

In addition to shortened lives, people in poverty are also more likely to be excluded from a quality of health experience available to those who are better off. The *General Household Survey* and the *Health Survey for England* are regular sources of information on morbidity and social circumstances. The *Health Survey for England* (Joint Health Surveys Unit 1997) indicates that a range of health factors and conditions are associated with social class, with men and women in poorer social classes more likely to have raised blood pressure and experience cardiovascular disorders than those in the highest social class. Similar patterns are evident in analyses of *General Household Survey* data. Benzeval's analysis of the *General Household Survey* data 1992 to 1994 shows that adults and children in the bottom two-fifths of the income distribution are much more likely to report a limiting long-standing illness than those at the top of the income distribution (Benzeval 1997). A small number of British studies have looked more directly at the relationship between income and health. Blaxter (1990), analysing data from the *Health and Lifestyles Survey*, found a clear relationship between income and health, with low-income groups experiencing higher morbidity and disability rates. Blaxter suggests that the apparent strong association between social class and health was primarily one of income and health.

While the evidence from large-scale morbidity and mortality research studies is important, it offers a one-dimensional and limited view of health exclusion in poverty. An additional and complementary view emerges from qualitative studies which have sought to record people's exclusion from good health. A Family Service Unit study of the experiences of sixty-five low-income families documented that poor health was a common experience. Over 65 per cent of the families interviewed reported poor health or disability among parents, and over 70 per cent among children (Cohen *et al.* 1992). Kempson's review of a number of studies of life on low income highlights that ill-health in poverty is associated with stress and the inability to meet the extra expenses associated with poor health and disability (Kempson 1996).

The evidence that low-income households have poorer health than their better-off counterparts is difficult to dispute. The evidence suggests a direct link (although we do not yet know whether it is a causal link) between poverty and poor health. Social inequalities in health appear to represent, at least in part, differences in income, as well as differences in social and economic circumstances, between social groups. Widening inequalities in health since the 1950s, often referred to as the 'health divide', appear to be related to relative trends in poverty (Wilkinson 1996). Although living standards over the century have risen overall, death and illness rates for the poor have not fallen as fast as death rates for the rich. Being healthy appears to require more than an absolute level of income to meet very basic needs. It appears to require a level of income that allows households to enjoy similar living standards and lifestyles to those of higher-income households (Quick and Wilkinson 1991).

Excluded from healthy lifestyles

Household income is a key health resource. First, it is the medium through which many economic and social resources reach household

members. Income influences both the social and economic circumstances within which people live and the way they live their lives. In
other words, income is a key determinant of people's lifestyles. Access
to healthy lifestyles through good housing, healthy food, a safe
environment, and to social and leisure facilities, depends, to a large
extent, on how much money is available to a household and on how
it is distributed within it. Focusing on poverty provides a way of
examining how one health hazard, low income, increases people's
exposure to other health hazards (Blackburn 1991). Numerous
studies document how financial poverty excludes households with
children from the healthy lifestyles advocated in health promotion
policies and from the living standards enjoyed by a large majority of
the population. These studies show how low income exposes
households to unhealthy living conditions, constrains their healthy
behaviour, subjects them to stress and distress, and is associated with
the development and continuation of health-damaging behaviours,
such as cigarette smoking.

Many low-income households with children live in housing
conditions that are incompatible with good health. Poor housing
conditions are experienced disproportionately by low-income
households (Arblaster and Hawtin 1993, Blackburn 1991). They are
less likely to own their own home and more likely to live in damp,
overcrowded homes that are poorly constructed and in need of repair.
Women and children bear the brunt of poor housing conditions. The
reasons are two-fold. First, they spend longer periods than men
within the home and thus are more likely to be exposed to the
hazards of poor housing. Second, women's relative economic
disadvantage compared to men means that female-headed households
find themselves least able to afford decent housing. Substandard
housing is also experienced disproportionately by Black and minority
ethnic households. Studies have highlighted that Black and minority
ethnic families are more likely than White families to be housed in
high-density areas in inner cities and to experience racial discrimination in the housing allocation and exchange systems if living in
public-sector rented accommodation (Luthera 1989). Unhealthy
conditions within the home are often compounded by poor external
environments and geographical locations which have poor community resources, such as childcare, education and leisure facilities.

Lack of choice about housing location may result in families being
housed away from the support structures available through kinship
and friendship networks. Good social support networks appear to be
important resources for good mental health, acting as buffers against

stress (Schwarzer and Leppin 1991). Caring for children and poverty are two experiences known to be associated with high levels of stress and mental distress (Graham 1993, Whelan 1993), yet it has been demonstrated that low-income households with children often have low social support resources (Oakley *et al.* 1994, Willmot 1987). Studies suggest that kinship and friendship networks are not only important sources of emotional support but that they can also be valuable sources of financial and material support to families (McKee 1987). For Black and minority ethnic groups, the stress associated with poverty may be further compounded by the daily experience of racism. Black people's accounts highlight that racial harassment is common and linked to poor heath and mental distress (Douglas 1996, Eyles and Donovan 1990).

Low household income constrains the health behaviour of many households. The adoption and maintenance of unhealthy behaviours and lifestyles by low-income groups has been of continuing concern among health promoters. Across a range of health behaviours, low-income households have less healthy lifestyles than their better-off counterparts. This is most clearly evident in, but not limited to, the food consumption patterns and expenditure patterns associated with low income. Low-income households appear to spend a higher proportion of their income on food and have diets that are higher in fats and sugar and lower in fibre than those of higher income groups (Ministry of Agriculture, Fisheries and Food 1989). A number of studies have examined food consumption and expenditure patterns in families with children, concluding that they consume unhealthy diets, not because of poor knowledge about the constituents of a healthy diet or unhealthy attitudes, but because they cannot afford to buy the foods that are considered important for good health (Cole-Hamilton 1988, Kempson 1996). Healthy foods are not only more expensive than unhealthy foods, but they are also less readily available to households who depend on local shopping facilities. Food availability is particularly an issue for Black and minority ethnic families. Traditional foods are often less readily available and more expensive than foods common to the diet of the White, majority population.

The daily food hardships and struggles of low-income households are reflected in a number of studies. These studies indicate that households cut back on food expenditure and consumption when money is short (NCH Action for Children 1994, Dallison and Lobstein 1995). Food costs, unlike housing and fuel costs, appear to be a flexible item in the household budget, on which expenditure can be decreased or increased, depending on how much money is available each week. Lack of money and poor availability of healthy foods combine to restrict the diets of low-income households. Kempson (1996), reviewing a number of studies of low-income living, concluded that low income 'leads to poor diets, with choices between eating healthy foods or having sufficient to eat'. A study of the eating patterns of low-income households with children, carried out by NCH Action for Children (1994), documents their food poverty: no parent or child who participated in a detailed nutritional study was eating a healthy diet as recommended by nutritionists for a healthy life. Moreover, one in five parents and one in ten children had gone without food in the last month because of lack of money. Similar findings were uncovered by a study of diet in pregnancy (Dallison and Lobstein 1995). This study uncovered that three-quarters of low-income pregnant women regularly missed meals, and over a third had diets that were seriously deficient in five or more vitamins and minerals.

Poor health in poverty is also associated with the development and continuation of health-damaging behaviours such as cigarette smoking. Cigarette smoking has increasingly become a habit associated with social disadvantage and poverty, as smoking rates among low-income groups have failed to decline as sharply as those of higher-income groups. Cigarette smoking rates are three times as high in social class V as social class I (Joint Health Surveys Unit 1997) and appear to increase as levels of social and material disadvantage increase (Marsh and MacKay 1994, Graham and Blackburn 1998). High smoking rates are reported in low-income households with children, particularly lone mother households (Marsh and MacKay 1994, Blackburn and Graham 1995).

Cigarette smoking appears to be closely linked to caring for children in difficult circumstances. Low-income households smoke more cigarettes and spend substantial proportions of their household budget on cigarettes (Townsend 1995). Graham's work (1996) on women's health work illustrates how health-damaging behaviours such as cigarette smoking are maintained against a background of caring in disadvantaged circumstances. Graham suggests that the smoking habits of low-income mothers are part of a 'broader lifestyle fashioned out of the needs and constraints of caring for children'. For women on low incomes, struggling with the relentless demands of caring in difficult circumstances, cigarette smoking provides a way of managing and diffusing stress. It is experienced not as a lifestyle choice but as a compromise to protect family health (Graham 1996).

Compromising health needs and health activities appears to provide a way of managing shortages of health resources, and lack of power and control in poverty. Several types of compromises can be discerned from parental accounts of caring for family health in poverty. First, caring on a low income often means compromising one health activity, for example healthy eating, in favour of another, such as providing warmth by paying fuel bills. Second, one person's health may be compromised to promote the health of another. Parents appear to compromise their own health, for example through smoking and cutting their own consumption of food, to promote the health of their children. Compromising health needs and health activities results in less health exclusion for some (often children) and more health exclusion for others (usually mothers). Seeking to understand how health behaviour is compromised on a low income highlights that unhealthy lifestyles are the outcome of a complex set of decisions that parents make in the face of poverty.

Excluded from health services provision

While there is little doubt that current resource allocation systems have gone a long way towards addressing major historical inequalities in health care, the evidence suggests that some social groups, including low-income households, still experience difficulties accessing health services. Although health services alone are not in themselves sufficient to address low-income households' exclusion from good health – this is dependent on a much broader range of social provision – they have a role to play in reducing the effects of health exclusion and promoting equality in health (NHS Centre for Reviews and Dissemination 1995). To reduce health exclusion, health services must, first, be accessible to those who need to use them and second, be provided in a form responsive to the needs of users.

The social distribution of poor health and illness described earlier in this chapter suggest that at any one time, low-income households are more likely than other groups to be caring for someone who is sick or disabled than better-off families. There is little doubt that low-income households absorb substantial amounts of health care resources and are heavy users of health services. But research studies of health service utilisation by low-income households suggest a mixed picture. On the one hand, there is evidence of under-utilisation of preventive services and concern that low-income households may fail to seek, or delay in seeking, help when someone is ill. Evidence suggests that low-income households with children are less likely than higher income households to use preventive services. For example, immunisation uptake rates, child health clinic attendances, and uptake rates for other preventive care has been found to be lower among low-income households (Marsh and Channing 1987, Gillam 1992, Reading *et al.* 1994). On the other hand, there is evidence of heavy use of some curative services by low-income households. Marsh and Channing (1987) found that general practitioner patients living in a deprived area had 60 per cent more hospital admissions and 75 per cent more casualty attendance than matched patients living in more 'endowed' areas.

Although further research is required, there is also evidence of some inequalities in patterns of treatment and care. For example, Ben-Shloma and Chaturvedi (1995) established that patients in disadvantaged areas were less likely to receive a coronary artery bypass graft than those living in more affluent areas. A survey examining mental health services for children also found inequalities in patterns of treatment. Kurtz *et al.* (1994) found that the need for care was positively associated with disadvantage but negatively associated with the availability of psychiatrists. Reading and Allen (1997) examined social inequalities in health and health visitors' work. They concluded that, even though greater health visitor time was provided to very disadvantaged caseloads, this did not compensate for the large differences in demands between affluent and disadvantaged caseloads.

Trying to untangle the reasons for inequalities and inequities in access to services, treatment and care is complex. The evidence suggests that a number of factors come in to play to exclude low-income households from using and receiving health service provision. These include the presence of material and social barriers, inequities in resource allocation and practitioner attitudes and perceptions. For some low-income households, material barriers to the use of preventive and curative health services remain. While some health authorities and trusts have sought to reduce geographical barriers to health care by maintaining local provision and providing outreach services in disadvantaged areas, some households find that the geographical location of services makes them difficult to use. There is some evidence that health services are more likely to be located in more affluent areas (Whitehead 1992). Recent health care reforms have led to the centralisation of some services, including acute hospital services. Travelling to access health care, when public transport is the main form of transport, places not only financial barriers, but also time and emotional barriers in the way of accessing health care. Pearson *et al.*'s research (1993) has illustrated the far-reaching effects that poor local availability of services can have on low-income households. Not only did attending GP surgeries, community health clinics and out-patient departments require travelling long distances, often by bus or taxi, they also involved substantial periods of time and required considerable creativity and skill in terms of providing care for other family members, such as children. Carers had to 'borrow' time and resources from others to get to appointments and to provide care for dependants left at home. This study illustrates that, for some households, in some circumstances, the costs (financial, time and social) may outweigh the perceived benefits of seeking care and treatment.

Although health care under the NHS is free at the point of delivery, user charges are on the increase, with charges for prescriptions, dental care and eye tests now in place. Although there is extensive evidence from the United States on the impact of user charges on utilisation of and access to health care, few British studies exist. Evidence from this small number of studies, however, suggests that the introduction of user charges in Britain is associated with reduced access to care for some individuals who are not exempt from charges. Ryan and Birch's (1991) analysis of increases in prescription charges and patient utilisation concluded that prescription charges have resulted in a reduction in utilisation among those who are not exempt from charges. Although some groups, including children and people in receipt of income support, are exempt from prescription charges, others are not. From April 1998, prescription charges increased to £5.80 per item, a twenty-nine-fold increase in charges since 1979. There is also concern over the introduction of charges for dental treatment and eye tests. It has been suggested that charges act as a deterrent to seeking help at an early stage. A study of the identification of glaucoma, an eye disease which is symptomatic in its early stages, suggests that there has been a significant reduction in referrals from opticians for glaucoma since the introduction of eye test charges in 1989 (Laidlaw *et al.* 1994). There is also concern about access to dental care. Pollack (1995) has suggested that charges discourage dentists from setting up practices in disadvantaged areas, where they are unlikely to make a good income.

Promoting equal and equitable access is dependent on making services socially and culturally acceptable. Improving the social and cultural acceptability of services to Black and minority ethnic groups is of paramount importance. When compared with other low-income households, Black and minority ethnic groups experience similar barriers to service use, and more. Language differences create considerable difficulties for some users in a service where the majority of care-givers are White and where the availability of link-workers and interpreters is patchy. The Smethwick Heart Action Programme, a locality-based research project set up to establish the health experiences and needs of Black and minority ethnic groups, highlighted how lack of interpreting services and racism in the health service had affected people's access to information and services. The study also suggested that stereotypical views among White practitioners (for example, about religious beliefs prohibiting women from taking physical exercise) can influence the availability of services (Douglas 1996).

Providing services in a form that meets the needs of disadvantaged households is key to proving inclusionary services. Blackburn (1993) suggests that many health practitioners fail to respond to low-income households in ways that address their poverty-related health needs. Although there is evidence of good practice, many practitioners have reactive styles of work concerned with individual behaviour change. As the earlier part of this chapter documents, poor health and unhealthy behaviour in poverty are a response to, and a consequence of the daily experience of, low-income living. Focusing on individual behaviour in isolation from its social context inflates the link with unhealthy lifestyles and fails to acknowledge the structural causes of poor health in poverty. It results in provision that incorporates material and social barriers to using services, and in services which fail to promote material and social support.

Failure to respond adequately to poverty and its consequences for health is associated with a number of factors. Legislation and policies have redefined roles in ways that have legitimated individualistic approaches and made it increasingly difficult to move towards proactive responses to poverty and health issues. Factors concerned with practitioners' attitudes to and knowledge about poverty are also responsible. Attitudes to household poverty and explanations about the causes of poor health in poverty are embodied in health care policies, strategies and methods of intervention. Practitioners appear to hold a variety of views about the causes and nature of poverty and its relationship to health. While some workers will operate with structural explanations of poverty, others may utilise more individualistic explanations, where individuals are seen as responsible for their own poverty and poor health (Popay *et al.* 1986, Becker 1988). Despite a renewed interest in poverty, health practitioners do not necessarily see what they do as related to poverty (Blackburn 1991). As a result, practice remains at the margins of poverty and health exclusion.

Tackling health exclusion in poverty: what role for practitioners?

It is important to recognise that tackling the health exclusion experienced by low-income households with children is dependent, largely, on tackling the structural causes of poverty and income inequality. This is dependent on a wide-ranging and radical restructuring of social and economic policies relating to employment, income maintenance, childcare and education (Benzeval *et al.* 1995). While it is important to recognise that health services can have little impact on the structural causes of poverty, the nature and form of service provision has an important bearing on how low-income families experience poor health in poverty. Health care practitioners have a central role to play, challenging policies that promote health exclusion and providing services that seek to assist families to avoid, mitigate and cope with the worst effects of poverty on health (Blackburn 1992).

It is important to recognise that there is no single or simple solution that can be adopted by health practitioners to reduce the health exclusion experienced by low-income households. Poverty and health exclusion are not experienced uniformly by individuals, social groups or across localities. Nor do practitioners' groups or organisations have similar levels of resources, remits or concerns. The details of strategies need to be worked out with individual communities, and within and across practitioner groups and organisations. Although there is no single blueprint for tackling health exclusion in poverty, there are a number of key points for practitioners that emerge from a review of the research on poverty and poor health.

The development and provision of services that respond to health exclusion in poverty are likely to depend on building an overt poverty perspective into health practice. Challenging negative practitioner attitudes to poverty and low-income users of services, and building up knowledge about the structural causes of poverty and poor health are central to this. Qualification and post-qualification education courses and staff development programmes must develop in ways that give practitioners the knowledge and skills to integrate a poverty and health exclusion perspective into everyday practice. Moreover, they must assist practitioners to develop and sharpen core skills: health profiling, providing preventive and alleviating responses, and working for social change.

The use of health profiling skills to monitor and disseminate information on poverty and poor health is central to developing proactive responses. Health profiling activities that can generate data about the extent of health exclusion in poverty, its nature and its causes are a vital tool to inform the development of services. While community health practitioners have been involved in health profiling activities for some time, health profiles do not necessarily contain information on health exclusion. In the light of likely policy developments to give primary health care practitioners, particularly community nurses, key roles in locality commissioning groups (DOH 1997), the development and fine-tuning of health profiling skills is paramount.

Even though there is now government acknowledgement in the Green Paper *Our Healthier Nation* that poverty and social exclusion are major causes of ill health (DOH 1998), there are no signs that there will be a radical restructuring of social and economic policies to reduce them in the near future. Assuming that health exclusion in poverty will continue to be an everyday reality for many low-income households, it is important that practitioners continue to develop strategies and services that assist households to avoid, mitigate and cope with health exclusion in poverty. Developing ways of working that acknowledge to families that they are not to blame for their poor health are important. This means respecting parental choices and recognising that parents are forced to compromise their own and their children's health in poverty. Key responses include those that seek to maximise household access to income (for example through tying welfare rights and health information together) and other important health resources (for example through food cooperatives and home safely equipment loan schemes). In the light of strong evidence that low-income households have poorer access to health services than better-off groups, it would seem that, as part of an ameliorative response, practitioners need to ensure that material, social and language barriers to using services are minimised. Given that there are likely to be few additional resources, responding to the excess of poor health found among low-income households requires directing resources to those whose needs are greatest and away from those whose needs are minimal (Billingham 1998). Health profiles are key resources to guide targeting and prioritisation.

At the same time, there is a need to maintain some sense of what can be achieved through responses that seek to challenge local and national policies that promote and maintain health exclusion. Health profile information and practitioner knowledge of the health experiences of low-income households are important tools for practitioners seeking to do this. Practitioners have an important role to play in sharing information with local communities who are mounting their own challenges against health exclusion and fighting for more responsive and equitable health and social provision. Many practitioners are members of trade unions and professional organisa- tions which adopt strong lobbying roles on social inequalities in health. Supporting these organisations and forming alliances with anti-poverty groups are further ways of challenging health exclusion.

So far, this chapter has focused on low-income households as victims of health exclusion, yet low-paid workers in the health service may themselves be part of the exclusionary system. The health service employs large numbers of workers in low-paid jobs with poor employment conditions. Campaigning for better pay and conditions for low-paid health service employees at national and local level is an important dimension of working to reduce health exclusion. Social change responses are largely dependent on working with other agencies. Improving unhealthy and unsafe housing environments is likely to depend on coordinated action across a number of agencies. The value of multi-agency work lies in its ability to move responses away from attempts to find individual solutions to problems that are rooted beyond the individual, and in its potential to deal with financial, health and social issues in an integrated way.

Conclusion

Poverty and income inequality continue to be major social issues in Britain. A rise in poverty levels, particularly among households with dependent children, has been accompanied by a deterioration in the living standards of poor households. Low income and poverty are major causes of health exclusion. This chapter has outlined three dimensions of health exclusion. Focusing on the experiences of households with children, it has documented how households in poverty are excluded from good health, healthy lifestyles and responsive health service provision.

The evidence that low-income households have poorer health than their better-off counterparts is difficult to dispute. The evidence suggests a direct link (although we do not yet know whether it is a causal link) between poverty and poor health. But being healthy appears to require more than an absolute level of income to meet very basic needs. It appears to require a level of income that allows households to enjoy similar living standards and participate in society in similar ways to higher-income households. The evidence suggests that low-income families experience a substandard quality of life relative to their better-off counterparts.

It is important to acknowledge that tackling health exclusion in poverty requires a radical restructuring of social and economic policy to reduce income inequalities and unemployment, and to promote better access to housing, education and childcare. At the same time, there is a need to maintain a sense of what front-line practitioners can do to reduce health exclusion in poverty. Community practitioners are uniquely placed to collect and disseminate information on poverty and health exclusion, and to use it to shape responses which help households to avoid and cope with the worst aspects of health exclusion and which challenge policies that promote and maintain health exclusion. Responding to poor health in poverty is the major challenge facing health professionals at the present time. There is growing evidence that some practitioners are building proactive responses to tackle health exclusion in poverty. However, an overwhelming conclusion arising out of the literature on professional practice is that there is still a long to go to refocus practice away from its overriding concern with individual behaviour towards responses that acknowledge the structural causes of health exclusion.

References

Arblaster, L. and Hawtin, M. (1993) *Health, Housing and Social Policy*, London: Socialist Health Association.

Becker, S. (1988) 'Poverty awareness', in S. Becker and S. MacPherson (eds) *Public Issues, Private Pain*, London: Social Services Insight.

Ben-Shloma, Y. and Chaturvedi, N. (1995) 'Access to health care provision in the UK: does where you live affect your chances of getting a coronary artery bypass graft?', *Journal of Epidemiology and Community Health*, 49, 43–7.

Benzeval, M. (1997) 'Health', in A. Walker and C. Walker (eds) *Britain Divided: The Growth of Social Exclusion in the 1980s and 1990s*, London: CPAG.

Benzeval, M., Judge, K. and Whitehead, M. (eds) (1995) *Tackling Inequalities in Health: An Agenda for Action*, London: King's Fund.

Billingham, K. (1998) 'Child health surveillance: the state of the art', in N. Spencer (ed.) *Progress in Community Child Health*, London: Churchill Livingstone.

Blackburn, C. (1991) *Poverty and Health: Working with Families*, Milton Keynes: Open University Press.

——(1992) 'Family poverty: what can health visitors do?', *Health Visitor*, 64, 11: 368–70.

——(1993) 'Making poverty a practice issue', *Health and Social Care*, 1, 297–305.

——(1996) 'Building a poverty perspective into health visiting practice', in P. Bywaters and E. McLeod (eds) *Working for Equality in Health*, London: Routledge.

Blackburn, C. and Graham, H. (1995) *Achieving Lifestyle Change: A Survey of Mothers on Income Support in Three Community NHS Trusts in the Midlands*, Coventry: Department of Applied Social Studies, University of Warwick.

Blaxter, M. (1990) *Health and Lifestyles*, London: Routledge.

Cohen, R., Coxall, J., Craig, G. and Sadiq-Sangster, A. (1992) *Hardship Britain: Being Poor in the 1990s*, London: CPAG.

Cole-Hamilton, I. (1988) 'Review of food patterns among low income groups', Report for the Health Education Council (unpublished).

Dallison, J. and Lobstein, T. (1995) *Poor Expectations: Poverty and Undernourishment in Pregnancy*, London: NCH Action for Children/ Maternity Alliance.

Department of Health (DOH) (1997) *The New NHS: Modern, Dependable*, London: The Stationery Office.

——(1998) *Our Healthier Nation: A Contract for Health*, London: The Stationery Office.

Department of Social Security (DSS) (1980) *Social Security Statistics*, London: HMSO.

——(1996) *Households Below Average Income: A Statistical Analysis 1979–1993/4*, London: HMSO.

——(1997) *Social Security Statistics*, London: The Stationery Office.

Douglas, J. (1996) 'Developing with Black and minority ethnic communities: health promotion strategies which address social inequalities', in P. Bywaters and E. McLeod (eds) *Working for Equality in Health*, London: Routledge.

Eyles, J. and Donovan, J. (1990) *The Social Effects of Health Policy*, Aldershot: Avebury.

Gillam, S. (1992) 'Provision of health promotion clinics in relation to population need: another example of the inverse care law', *British Journal of General Practice*, 42, 54–6.

Goldblatt, P. (1990) (ed.) *Longitudinal Study: Mortality and Social Organisations 1971–1981*, OPCS Series No. 6, London: HMSO.

Goodman, A. and Webb, S. (1994) *For Richer for Poorer: The Changing Distribution of Income in the United Kingdom, 1961–91*, London: Institute for Fiscal Studies.

Graham, H. (1993) *Hardship and Health in Women's Lives*, Hemel Hempstead: Harvester Wheatsheaf.

——(1996) 'Researching women's health work: a study of the lifestyles of mothers on income support', in P. Bywaters and E. McLeod (eds) *Working for Equality in Health*, London: Routledge.

Graham, H. and Blackburn, C. (1998) 'The socio-economic patterning of health and smoking behaviour among mothers with young children on income support', *Sociology of Health and Illness*, 20, 2: 215–40.

Joint Health Surveys Unit (1997) *Health Survey for England 1995*, London: The Stationery Office.

Kempson, E. (1996) *Life on a Low Income*, York: Joseph Rowntree Foundation.

Kurtz, Z., Thornes, R. and Wolkind, S. (1994) *Services for the Mental Health of Children and Young People in England: A National Review*, London: Maudsley Hospital and South Thames (West) Regional Health Authority.

Laidlaw, D., Bloom, P., Hughes, A., Sparrow, J. and Marmion V. (1994) 'The sight test fee: effect of ophthalmology referrals and rate of glaucoma detection', *British Medical Journal*, 309, 634–6.

Lister, R. (1990) *The Exclusive Society: Citizenship and the Poor*, London: CPAG.

——(1997) *Citizenship: Feminist Perspectives*, Basingstoke: Macmillan.

Luthera, M. (1989) 'Race, community, housing and the state – a historical overview', in A. Bhat *et al.* (eds) *Britain's Black Population*, Aldershot: Gower.

Marsh, A. and MacKay, S. (1994) *Poor Smokers*, London: Policy Studies Institute.

Marsh, G. and Channing, D. (1987) 'Comparison in use of health services between a deprived and an endowed area', *Archives of Diseases in Childhood*, 62, 392–6.

McKee, L. (1987) 'Households during unemployment: the resourcefulness of the unemployed', in J. Brannon and G. Wilson (eds) *Give and Take in Families*, London: Allen and Unwin.

Ministry of Agriculture, Fisheries and Food (1989) *Household Food Consumption and Expenditure, Annual Report of the National Food Survey 1987*, London: HMSO.

NCH Action for Children (1994) *Poverty and Nutrition Survey*, London: NCH Action for Children.

NHS Centre for Reviews and Dissemination (1995) *Review of the Research on the Effectiveness of Health Service Interventions to Reduce Variations in Health*, CRD Report 3, York: NHS Centre for Reviews and Dissemination.

Oakley, A., Rigby, A. and Hickey, D. (1994) 'Life stress, support and class inequality', *European Journal of Public Health*, 4, 81–91.

Pearson, M., Dawson, C., Moore, H. and Spence, S. (1993) 'Health on borrowed time? Prioritising and meeting needs in low-income households', *Health and Social Care*, 1, 1: 45–54.

Pollack, A. (1995) 'Privatisation by stealth?', *Health Visitor*, 68, 3: 98–9.

Popay, J., Dhooge, Y. and Shipman, C. (1986) *Unemployment and Health: What Role for Health and Social Services?* Research Report No. 3, London: Health Education Council.

Quick, A. and Wilkinson, R. (1991) *Income and Health*, London: Socialist Health Association.

Reading, R. and Allen, C. (1997) 'The impact of social inequalities in child health on health visitors' work', *Journal of Public Health Medicine*, 19, 4: 424–30.

Reading, R., Colver, A., Openshaw, S. and Jarvis, S. (1994) 'Do interventions that improve immunisation uptake also reduce social inequalities in uptake?', *British Medical Journal*, 308, 1142–4.

Room, G. (1995) *Beyond the Threshold*, London: The Polity Press.

Ryan, M. and Birch, S. (1991) 'Charging for health care: evidence on the utilisation of NHS prescribed drugs', *Social Science and Medicine*, 33, 6: 681–7.

Schwarzer, R. and Leppin, A. (1991) 'Social support and health: a theoretical and empirical overview', *Journal of Social and Personal Relationships*, 8, 99–127.

Townsend, J. (1995) 'The burden of smoking', in M. Benzeval, K. Judge and M. Whitehead (eds) *Tackling Inequalities in Health: An Agenda for Action*, London: King's Fund.

Walker, A. (1997) 'Introduction: the strategy of inequality', in A.Walker and C. Walker (eds) *Britain Divided: The Growth of Social Exclusion in the 1980s and 1990s*, London: CAPG.

Whelan, C. (1993) 'The role of social support in mediating the psychological consequences of economic stress', *Sociology of Health and Illness*, 15, 1: 87–101.

Whitehead, M. (1992) *The Health Divide*, London: Health Education Council.

Wilkinson, R. (1996) *Unhealthy Societies: The Afflictions of Inequality*, London: Routledge.

Willmot, P. (1987) *Friendship Networks and Social Support*, London: Policy Studies Institute.

Woodroffe, C., Glickman, M., Barker, M. and Power, C. (1993) *Children, Teenagers and Health: The Key Data*, Buckingham: Open University Press.

3 Whose business?

Social welfare and managerial calculation

John Clarke

The reconstruction of the welfare state in the UK has brought about changes in the form and role of the state and changes in what welfare means. This chapter explores the changing character of social welfare in the context of new ways of organising, providing and delivering welfare. The chapter does not focus explicitly or exclusively on health care. Rather, it examines the intersection between changes in organising health services and the changing form and role of the state in social welfare more generally. Drawing on work elsewhere (Clarke *et al.* 1994, Clarke and Newman 1997), I suggest that the *managerialisation* of state welfare is a significant development with consequences that reach far beyond the claims of making publicly provided services more 'businesslike'. Indeed, the chapter will address some of the ways in which the development of managerialism has had perverse consequences for the welfare of the public, despite widespread claims of increased efficiency in service provision.

Towards a new welfare system

The break-up of the old welfare state has led to many commentators describing the process as one of 'fragmentation', an idea particularly associated with conceptions of the transition from Fordism to post-Fordism (Burrows and Loader 1994). However, by itself the idea of fragmentation leaves open the issue of how such fragments are integrated – or coordinated (see Hoggett 1996). In addressing the reconstruction of the welfare state, we have found it useful to describe these movements as *dispersal* rather than fragmentation. The idea of dispersal makes it possible to talk about these processes as being linked to strategic political calculation, rather than treating them as inevitable occurrences (linked to processes of globalising change) or dealing with public sector restructurings as a necessary imitation of corporate sector organisational innovations. The idea of dispersal also draws attention to the ways in which 'agency' is being distributed by and from the centre to organisations and other social actors. We have seen the state delegating its authority to subaltern organisations that are then empowered to act – given degrees of conditional 'freedom to manage' their affairs and conduct their business. Processes of decentralisation, devolution and delegation within and between organisations have been recurrent features of the process of reconstructing the welfare state (see Birchall *et al.* 1995). The outcomes of these processes of dispersal may well be experienced as fragmentation and the disintegration of services and institutions. This has certainly been a central issue argued over in the reconstruction of the National Health Service (for example, Mohan 1995). But to describe the effects is not the same thing as identifying the processes that have produced such effects. The idea of dispersal, then, opens up questions about the relations of power that both underpin and act through these processes, not least the means by which the 'centre' – in this case central government – attempts to maintain command while distributing some forms of power to the 'periphery'.

These processes of dispersal underlie many of the changes in health and social care in particular (see, *inter alia*, Langan 1998b, Pinkney 1998). The shift during the 1990s towards more 'mixed economies' of welfare provision, with a declining role in direct provision for public agencies and an expanded role for commercial- and voluntary-sector based organisations, embodied forms of dispersal. So too did the movements towards market-like mechanisms for coordinating the provision of services both between and within organisations, together with the construction of purchaser/provider or client/contractor distinctions (Walsh 1995). At the same time, claims to be moving provision towards more 'needs-led' forms of organisation also reflect ideas of dispersing power – 'empowering' users (or customers) or those representing them in contracting arrangements (Clarke 1997). As we will see later in this chapter, such 'empowerment' in the context of dispersal has always been conditional, partial, and often contradictory. At the same time, it is also important to see the way in which these processes of dispersal have multiplied the number of organisations, and the number of places within, between and on the edges of organisations at which decisions about service provision might take place. As parents, clients, users, patients, customers become 'empowered'; as schools, hospitals, GPs, social services departments are 'set free' from old bureaucratic controls; and as units within such organisations are given devolved budgetary and other decision-making powers, so there has been a proliferation of decision-making possibilities within a new welfare system. This chapter explores some of the consequences of those changes and is particularly directed to the question of what imperatives, tensions and contradictions are embedded in this new system.

One strong strand in the reconstruction of the welfare state through these processes of dispersal has been the attempt to *depoliticise* the field of decision-making by turning many decisions about the alignment of resources and needs into matters of 'operational management'. Paul Hoggett has argued that 'there is a danger that naturalistic assumptions may guide policy makers and organizational analysts which obscure how the boundaries of the "operational" and the "strategic" are in fact socially constructed' (1996: 19). This constructed distinction between strategic and operational decisions has underpinned the oscillation between what Harrison *et al.* (1992) called 'hands-off and hands-on management', where the nominal line between policy and operational management is more honoured in the breach than the observance. In the NHS, the Prison Service, social care and education, governments have consistently attempted to distance themselves from crises and controversies by insisting that these are not questions of policy or the responsibility of ministers. For example, the perceived crisis arising from the overload of accident and emergency facilities in 1996 was identified by ministers as 'an issue for local management'. Langan (1998c: 25) suggests this process can be seen as an effort 'to centralise credit and diffuse blame'. Nevertheless, what is striking about these attempts to depoliticise controversial issues is the relatively limited success they have achieved. Even where ministers and their representatives have attempted to shift responsibility to managers, the dominant public perception seems to have remained that these matters are the proper business of government, with the result that they are consistently repoliticised in an oscillating sequence of accusations and denials.

Such developments have been visible in the creation of Civil Service Agencies and in the shift of public services to more autonomous organisational forms which limit democratic processes of accountability (grant maintained schools, hospital trusts, etc.). It has also been a core feature of the 'intermediate' institutions that have supplanted some of the traditional functions of local government, such as TECs, HATs and other quasi-public bodies. Such bodies embody the belief that the combination of 'men of good sense' – what John Stewart (1993) has called the 'new magistracy' – and managers who have been 'empowered' to manage will produce more efficient services, freed from the dogma of politics. The argument that this process has produced a 'democratic deficit' is contested by the claim that the change has led to greater levels of transparency of decision-making, and by enhanced patterns of direct accountability to the consumers of public services (Stewart 1993, Waldegrave 1993). Such debates suggest that the *forms of legitimation* of the new system remain contested issues. In particular, there continue to be arguments over whether 'good management' can be an adequate substitute for 'good government'.

Becoming businesslike? The rise of managerialism

In part, the new role for management in social welfare derived from the New Right's ideological insistence on the innate superiority of the market over the state as a means of allocating resources. In their view, managers inhabited the world of market action and were the natural carriers of its entrepreneurialism and dynamism. They could provide the full gamut of 'good business practices' which organisations in the public sector needed to learn. This imagery of management was often concerned with old-fashioned virtues of organisational coordination: the 'hard-headed' control of costs in the pursuit of greater efficiency, not least through intensified labour productivity (Mohan 1995). But this imagery of management also drew on the more dynamic celebration of the manager-as-hero being articulated in the 'new' managerialism, particularly in those new conceptions of the manager as leader and corporate culture shaper, inspiring the unending pursuit of quality and excellence (Clarke and Newman 1993a, Pollitt 1993, Flynn 1994). Both old and new versions of managerialism, however, centred on one essential precondition for 'transforming' the dull professional bureaucracies of social welfare into modern organisations – the establishment or enlargement of 'the right to manage'. Such legitimations of the 'natural' desirability of management as the obvious way of running organisations were reflected in the increasing use of the phrase 'well managed' to describe successful organisations. They were also sustained by contrasts drawn between management and the forms of organisational coordination associated with the old welfare state. The virtues of managers were compared with the failings of bureaucrats, professionals and politicians. So, where bureaucrats were rule-bound, inward-looking and inert, managers were innovative, externally oriented and dynamic. Where professionals were paternalistic, developed mystiques of expertise to conceal and protect their power, and were self-regulating, managers were customer-centred, created transparent organisations and were tested in the 'real world' of the market-place. Finally, where politicians were dogmatic, interfering and changeable, managers were realists, capable of taking a strategic view and, as long as they were given the 'freedom to manage', were able to deliver on the promise that they would 'do the right thing' (Clarke 1998a).

The reconstruction of the welfare system has involved both managerialism and managerialisation. Managerialism is an ideology that legitimates claims to power, especially the 'right to manage', legitimated as necessary to achieve greater efficiency in pursuing organisational and social objectives (see Pollitt 1993, chapter 1). Managerialism is also a calculative framework that organises knowledge about organisational goals and the means of achieving them. It is usually structured around an internal calculus of efficiency (inputs–outputs) and an external calculus of competitive positioning within a field of market relations (Newman 1998). However, managerialism is also a series of overlapping discourses that articulate different – even conflicting – propositions about how to manage and what is to be managed. So different forms of managerialism focus on 'leadership', 'strategy', 'quality' and so on to produce a complex and shifting field of managerial knowledge (see Pollitt 1993, Flynn 1994).

Managerialisation is a process of establishing managerial authority over corporate resources (whether these are material, human or symbolic) and corporate decision-making. It is also a process of establishing the calculative frameworks of managerialism. These define the terms and conditions of decision-making. The objective of managerialisation is to embed these frameworks as the forms of knowledge that govern patterns of internal and external relationships. Finally, managerialisation is a process of creating forms of 'managing' and types of managers. There have been three main forms of 'managing' visible in the restructuring of social welfare: 'real managers'; 'hybrids'; and a 'dispersed managerial consciousness'. The most obvious indicator of the impact of managerialism in social welfare is the rapid growth in the number of people who are employed as 'managers': that is, they occupy posts explicitly defined as 'management'. These managers are either 'imports' or 'converts':

the former are brought in from elsewhere; the latter are manufac-
tured 'in-house' through management training or development
programmes and making a career shift to a clearly identified
managerial role (in a context where organisational careers are
increasingly becoming defined in managerial rather than professional
terms). Although such numbers may be the most obvious indicator of
managerialisation, the other two forms of managing may be of equal
importance. The 'hybrid' form has become widespread in what were
formerly bureau-professional organisations providing welfare
services. 'Hybrid' is a convenient way of describing the complex
processes of incorporating professional workers into managerialised
roles, characteristically through processes of devolution and
delegation (Clarke and Newman 1993b, see also Ferlie *et al.* 1996).
Clinical directors, ward managers and fundholding practices in the
NHS; headteachers under Local Management of Schools; care
management in personal social services; devolved operational
management in policing all rest on the construction of articulations
between professional and managerial modes of coordination. Such
'hybrids' evoke a complex of motivations. On the one hand, they
mobilise 'service values' or professional commitments to motivate the
engagement with corporate management. At the same time, they
require that these commitments are subjected to the discipline of
accepting the 'realities' and 'responsibilities' of corporate management. In the process, it is possible to trace different sorts of
experiences of becoming a 'hybrid'. Some people have become
'empowered', enthusiastic converts to the world of management.
Others remain 'covert professionals', using new possibilities of power
and authority to preserve, deliver or even enhance services. Finally,
some become disenchanted 'cynics' – finding 'management speak' a
sham behind which their major task is that of managing decline.

Managerialisation is inextricably tied to other tendencies in the
remaking of the welfare state in Britain: the political initiatives of
neo-conservatism; the pursuit of the three E's ('economy, efficiency
and effectiveness') of fiscal responsibility in public spending, as well
as having a specific place in the policies of social care, health care,
education and so on (Clarke *et al.* 1994). But managerialisation is
also an independent process in its own right – embedded in
management education and development, private and public sector
management writing, and the roles of agencies such as the Audit
Commission, the Office for Public Management and the Local
Government Management Board, as well as the initiatives of specific
local authorities and agencies. Organisational reform, reconstruction

and re-engineering have attained epidemic proportions. Waves of restructurings, cultural change programmes, newly devolved and decentralised systems and varieties of performance management have washed over the welfare system. In these processes of reform, managerialism challenged the 'old ways' of running things in central and local government. Local political representation was marginalised by the shift of public resources to non-elected agencies and quangos, while being more tightly circumscribed by expanded central government control of both policy and resources. Methods of bureaucratic administration were challenged by the promise of a more dynamic and entrepreneurial approach to managing organizations. Professionalism was placed on the defensive by the assertion of customer-centred models of provision and the fragmentation of professional and bureaucratic tasks. This challenge was driven by the belief that professionals and street-level bureaucrats could be disciplined by devolved managerial systems that installed new responsibilities for resource control (Langan and Clarke 1994).

The legitimacy of managerialism, like that of bureau-professionalism, is also associated with its internal knowledge-base and the sciences and technologies from which this is derived. Bureau-professionalism offered the pursuit of the public good based on the application of forms of expert power that were service-specific. These were 'substantive' forms of knowledge about particular sorts of needs and interventions. By contrast, managerialism promises the best use of public resources based on the deployment of calculative power. The knowledge of managerialism is 'universalist', applicable to all organisations rather than substantive or service-specific. It is presented as a rationality which transcends the differences of services or sectors. The rationalism of managerialism thus appears as a non-partisan (and depoliticised) framework within which choices can be made. Competing values can be reduced to alternative sets of options, and the costs associated with them can be assessed in terms of their contribution to the organisation's performance. Competing values are thus subjected to a 'rational' analysis that claims to stand outside of the partisan demands of the different 'interest groups' that make up the organisation. While different professional or occupational groups may pursue their parochial interests, management stands for the organisation's best interests (see, for example, Green and Armstrong's discussion of 'bed management', 1995). The calculative frameworks of managerialism thus provide a foundation for enacting new logics of rationing, targeting and priority setting. The scientific knowledges which they deploy position managers as neutral and impersonal. Managers can be trusted: they are not part of the wars between different political, occupational or other factional interests.

As a consequence, the rational/technical character of managerial knowledge offers the promise of resolving two different forms of 'chaos'. The first is the chaos that characterised the old welfare system – the irrationality of *unmanaged* processes in which the decision-making of 'street level bureaucrats' could not be controlled, and in which bureaucratic control mechanisms proliferated. Managerialism promises to impose a rationalised order on this chaos. The second promise of managerialism is that of coping with the complexities and uncertainties of the modern world – the 'chaos of the new' – through the quasi-scientific techniques of strategic management and the capacity to 'manage change' in turbulent times. Where bureaucracies adapt slowly and in a rather ramshackle fashion, creating new rules and functions to cope with new situations within a framework of getting by and making do, managerialism promises to *organise* the irrational and bring order to chaos. Only management can secure organisational survival and success in the face of an unstable, unpredictable and hostile environment (this issue is developed further in Clarke 1998b).

The changing organisational landscape

At the core of these changes has been the view that there is no reason why, if 'set free', managers of public organisations should not be able to match the accomplishments of private sector ones – especially in terms of gains in economy, efficiency and effectiveness (Birchall *et al.* 1995). There is, of course, a variety of problems about just what setting free means in this context, but the overall pattern of the changes has had profound consequences for the relationship between the internal and external environments of organisations. The most obvious one is that organisations have been driven to become more attentive and adaptive to their 'business environments' – responding to their customers, competitors, contractors, collaborators and so on. But these changes have also had the effect of installing what might be thought of as essential dimensions of the external environment within the internal structures and cultures of the organisation.

The starting-point for this was the creation of 'quasi-markets' (Le Grand and Bartlett 1993) involving forms of contracting relationship, from the introduction of Compulsory Competitive Tendering onwards, which have had the consequence of making organisations think of themselves as businesses and as having to learn how to be 'business like' (Hoggett 1996). One central issue has been the growing significance of resource management. During the 1980s financial accounting came to provide the dominant calculating framework for organisational decision-making in many, if not all, public services. The finance department rose in organisational status and power as a consequence. This change was the direct effect of the primacy given to 'economy' in the three E's, together with the fact that finance departments were the possessors of privileged – and organisationally valued – knowledges (Cochrane 1994: 147–9). This shift was, however, only a precursor to the much more significant process by which everyone (at least everyone in managerial positions) was expected to be 'financially responsible' by the 1990s. The processes of devolution and decentralisation multiplied the numbers of budget centres and budget-holders and spread 'budgetary consciousness' far and wide within organisations.

Such changes are, naturally, associated with a number of organisational tensions and conflicts. For example, they multiply the numbers of people who feel aggrieved about the size of their budgets. They establish groups of managerial resisters (those who didn't join to manage budgets) and enthusiasts (those who would like more freedom to manage their budgets creatively). They set in play hostilities between the finance department (possessors of 'real' knowledge) and devolved units (amateurs, or at least those who don't believe the finance department) which focus around the form and availability of information and the reconciliation of central and local information. These changes create a new discourse of 'trust' – or the lack thereof – within organisations. This was powerfully exemplified in the problems associated with the Community Care reform objectives of devolving budgets and purchasing power to front line 'care managers' (Audit Commission 1992, Langan and Clarke 1994). Once such changes have taken place, they have the effect of internalising what were previously external disciplines, controls and ways of thinking. As managers take possession of budgets, so they begin to think of themselves as 'owners'. This is clearly intentional (after all, management texts endlessly talk about the importance of creating 'ownership'), but such ownership may be less straightforward than is imagined. Possessiveness accelerates the centrifugal forces in organisations – exacerbating tendencies towards fragmentation. It also creates new patterns of internal competitiveness and resource conflicts as units strive to protect or enhance their budgets – and look to the new discourses of being businesslike to justify their claims.

In the process, the organisation itself becomes a 'competitive environment', characterised by new forms of internal conflict. It is important to stress 'new forms' here, since I have no wish to erect a nostalgic view of old organisational regimes being conflict-free zones, especially where resources were concerned. But what has changed is the way such conflicts are structured, the forms in which they take place, and the languages in which they are conducted. Most of the public sector reforms of the last decade have aimed to create internal markets or funding regimes which produce inter-organisational competitiveness (within certain constraints). So provider organisations are driven to compete for either customers or contracts on the basis of cost, quantity and (to a marginal extent) quality. Such external competitiveness is closely linked, however, to new intra-organisational competition as units or departments within the organisation struggle to claim the right to 'their' income. Such effects pose major issues about organisational integration for both corporate and local managements, in particular the question of what it is that holds the structure together beyond the 'quasi-contractual' arrangements. There has been a range of attempts to promote corporate cultures through the development of mission statements, corporate imagery and the like. Such developments often involve an uncomfortable attempt to use the symbolism of the contemporary business world (the rhetorics of efficiency, quality, excellence, investing in people, etc.) to re-present the organisation. We might note, in passing, the relative 'emptiness' of such corporate cultural statements, such that being businesslike seems to take precedence over the business. The language and symbolism often float free of the specific cluster of purposes, values and practices of the organisation (see Cutler and Waine 1994, on the adoption of 'general management').

At the same time as reforms have made organisations more attentive to their 'external environments', there have also been changes which have made organisational boundaries more permeable – and more susceptible to confusion between the inside and the outside. Perhaps the best example of this is to be found in the development of new types of inter-organizational partnerships which involve high levels of interdependence (see, for example, Huxham 1996). Historically, patterns of joint working or collaboration have tended to be accomplished at 'arm's length' through joint committees, boards, working groups, etc., established with representation from different agencies, reporting back for decisions to be made by the separate agencies. In such conditions, organisational 'integrity' was relatively well protected by formal mechanisms of separation. However, the changing pressures and possibilities of public sector organisations have made moves beyond such arm's length relationships a possible pattern of organisational development. There have been increasing possibilities for and pressures towards jointly resourced and jointly controlled activities or towards two or more partners creating a new – semi-autonomous – agency. Successful partnerships seem to depend on the surrendering of elements of organisational integrity and independence, but in the process this blurs the demarcation of inside and outside (Kanter 1994). Such changes pose problems for organisations around the tension between developing new 'flexible' forms of working interdependently and the pressure to maintain integrity and control in pursuit of their own 'core business'. Such tensions are visible, for example, in the problematic relationships between health and social services agencies in the development of community care, where attempts to create collaborative working run in the face of different (indeed possibly divergent) organisational, professional, managerial and economic concerns of the different agencies.

A second dimension along which the boundary between the internal and external worlds has become more blurred – or fluid – is the impact of processes of dispersal on the internal order of organisations. Increasingly, some sections of the organisation come to form part of the environment of other sections of the organisation while still, of course, being inside the organisation. This is most visible in the introduction of 'internal markets', in-house trading units and relationships, and purchaser/provider or client/contractor relationships within single agencies. In such circumstances, relationships which had been internal – and integrated through collegial or hierarchical mechanisms – have become 'quasi-external', and integrated through forms of contracting for services (for example, Local Management of Schools and the changing place of local authority education departments; or the shift to a purchasing relationship for central support services). In the tension between fragmentation and integration, this set of processes creates units with a double status – both inside and outside simultaneously – and enmeshed in multiple and often conflicting modes of integration. Thus, as *insiders*, units are likely to remain subject to (at least vestiges of) collegial and/or hierarchical modes of integration, while as *outsiders* they are increasingly subject to quasi-contractual relationships. For example, the development of the purchaser/provider split in local authority social services departments overlaid contractual relationships on what had historically been collegial/professional relationships (between different social work sections and specialisms), interprofessional relationships (between social workers and others such as occupational therapists, home care workers, etc.) and hierarchical/departmental structures of the organisation.

Nobody's business? Social welfare and managerialism

The pursuit of more economic and efficient welfare provision through managerialism has involved a range of strategies. Rationing has become a more visible and more significant process, ranging from the definition of health priorities to the requirement for local authorities to define those 'in need' of support through personal social services in both the Children Act of 1989 and the NHS and Community Care Act of 1990 (Langan 1998a). The wider political agenda of targeting welfare benefits and services has been reflected in new organisational forms of discretionary judgement, to be exercised in the balancing of needs and resources. The concern with targeting welfare provision has been closely tied to arguments about the need for greater efficiency, for example in the claims that universal benefits and services are fundamentally wasteful of resources and unnecessary in an affluent and privatised society. Targeting has created an extension of means testing for a variety of benefits and services in the place of access as of right. Although this has been most visible in the movement away from insured benefits to income support in the income maintenance system, it is also a strand in community care, education (as school provision narrows to the core curriculum), access to transport and leisure facilities, and aspects of health care. In the process, there are significant transfers of cost (both economic and social) out of the welfare system. The expectation that needs will be met by other means makes people 'independent' of the state in demanding ways, involving what Craig (1998) has called the 'privatisation of human misery'. At the same time, such policies have been legitimated on the basis of concentrating resources on the most needy. So, in addition to means testing, other forms of evaluation have come to occupy a significant place in the new welfare system. These have revived older debates about the relationship between need and moral worth – ranging from the 'undeserving' character of lone mothers to the denial of health resources to those who 'don't look after themselves' or are a 'bad investment' (Langan 1998c). Sarah Nettleton, among others, has drawn attention to the ways in which 'lifestyle' criteria are embedded in the new health paradigm (1996). The same paradigm also involves shifts of 'responsibility' outwards from the welfare system to individuals, who are expected (or enabled, or empowered) to 'manage' their own health needs.

The managerialisation of public services has attempted to resolve the contradictions between rising need and shrinking resources by turning this into a management problem – the production of 'more for less'. As a result, one of the dominant tasks for public sector management has become the management of demand. Where demand incurs costs (rather than being the reward for finding 'new business'), organisations find themselves enmeshed in gate-keeping as well as rationing processes. Such activities range from persuading the public to use a service less (visible in GP home visits, for example), through using charging as a filter, to redirecting users by redefining their needs. The most visible example of this last practice has been the redirection of patients to Accident and Emergency departments that are outside of the contracting process. These same issues are also at stake in the organisational task of defining 'core business'. This further involves each organisation (rather than service) in deciding what are not its corporate priorities. In this situation, there is a real danger that some needs will become 'nobody's business'.

The quasi-market mechanism and the accompanying division between purchasers and providers has used the imitation of market competition to drive down costs in 'provider' organisations as they compete for contracts. Since purchasing agencies possess limited funding, this tends to place the cost of contracting services as the dominant priority. This, in turn, sets the agenda for provider agencies, unless they can define themselves as providing a 'niche' service which carries a financial premium. As well as instilling cost consciousness, the competitive mechanism has other effects; for example, through the way competitors strive to control the conditions which will affect their costs (Le Grand and Bartlett 1993, Salter 1993, Mackintosh 1995, Cutler and Waine 1997). As Cutler and Waine have argued, however, the assumption that 'low cost' is a desirable organisational objective is far from straightforward: 'it ignores the question of how such "low costs" are achieved and...their possible implications for deterioration in levels and conditions of employment' (1997: 7). In these market-imitating processes, organisations increasingly have to calculate what or who constitutes a legitimate demand on their resources. They must also make choices about collaboration and partnership with a view to sharing burdens or increasing resources. They must also make calculations about the transfer of costs to other people's budgets. In these conditions, what might be called 'boundary management' has become an increasingly significant managerial task.

Boundary management is significant for relations between organisations. For example, it has been highly visible in the arguments about the long-term care needs of the elderly. The service and organisational boundaries between the NHS and social services have seen much action around the definition of needs and the allocation of responsibility for meeting them (Vickridge 1995). Julia Twigg has traced some of these realignments in her analysis of 'the social bath' (1997). She suggests that the provision of bathing is positioned 'across the principal fault line of community care: that between the medical and the social' (ibid.: 212). She argues that the 'social bath' is 'defined in negative terms: the sort of bath that the community nursing service does *not* provide' (ibid.) – that is, the 'social bath' is not a 'medical bath', and this signals its lower status and lower priority. She suggests that the positioning of care needs between medical and social care enmeshes them in overlapping definitions of public and private realms and allocations of cost and responsibility:

> The broad distinction between free health care and self-funded or means tested social care has become increasingly sharp in Britain as local authorities have moved towards charging for the principal services of community care – home, day and respite care – previously provided free or on a varying but nearly always non-commercial basis. The division between health and social care is increasingly a division between care that is free to the individual and that which has to be funded from his or her own purse.
>
> (ibid.: 214).

The process of boundary management is also an inter-sectoral matter, through attempts to manage 'creaming' and 'dumping' strategies in relation to good and bad risks (and their associated costs). Other inter-sectoral issues involve the transfer of costs via contracting-out provision: for example, exploiting the lower cost or even free labour available to voluntary sector organisations. Less visibly, inter-sectoral boundary management involves transfers between the formal – or organised – sectors of public provision and the informal world of the household. This process has been extensively discussed in relation to social care and to a lesser extent in relation to health care. In the latter, the most obvious example has been the achievement of faster hospital 'throughput' by transferring convalescence to the home setting. But it also applies to other 'efficiency gains' in state welfare provision. Education has increasingly come to rely on supplementation from familial resources: paying for extra-curricular provision; fund-raising for school budgets, and using parental labour more intensively both within the curriculum (for example, listening to children read) and in school management (in governing bodies and fund-raising). Reductions in the benefit levels and the increase in means testing for benefits and some services transfer the costs of living from public to private resources, such that households use up savings, practise better 'household management', or go into debt.

These issues suggest that the pursuit of organisational efficiency in social welfare has involved complex processes of cost transfer. One central way of achieving new levels of organisational efficiency has been to 'externalise' the costs of welfare, passing them on to other organisations, other services or other sectors. In particular, we have seen the 'privatisation' of some of the costs of social welfare. This means of pursuing efficiency generates a peculiar paradox. While welfare-providing organisations become increasingly efficient, their means of becoming efficient may add to (rather than reduce) the social problems and levels of need to which the state is asked to respond. The 'not our business' calculus of efficiency may improve organisational performance at the same time as diminishing the welfare of the public as a whole.

References

Audit Commission (1992) *The Community Revolution: Personal Social Services and Community Care*, London: HMSO.

Birchall, I., Pollitt, C. and Putnam, K. (1995) 'Freedom to manage? The experience of NHS Trusts, grant-maintained schools and voluntary transfers of public housing', paper to the UK Political Studies Association Annual Conference, York, April.

Burrows, R. and Loader, B. (eds) (1994) *Towards a Post-Fordist Welfare State?* London: Routledge.

Clarke, J. (1997) 'Capturing the customer? Consumerism and social welfare', *Self, Agency and Society*, 1, 1: 55–73.

——(1998a) 'Doing the right thing? Managerialism and social welfare', in P. Abbott (ed.) *The Sociology of the Caring Professions*, London: Taylor and Francis (second edition).

——(1998b) 'Thriving on chaos: managerialism and social welfare', in J. Carter (ed.) *Postmodernity and the Fragmentation of Social Welfare*, London: Routledge.

Clarke, J., Cochrane, A. and McLaughlin, E. (eds) (1994) *Managing Social Policy*, London: Sage.

Clarke, J. and Newman, J. (1993a) 'The right to manage: a second managerial revolution?', *Cultural Studies*, 7, 3: 427–41.

——(1993b) 'Managing to survive: dilemmas of changing organisational forms in the public sector', in N. Deakin and R. Page (eds) *The Costs of Welfare*, Aldershot: Avebury.

——(1997) *The Managerial State: Power, Politics and Ideology in the Remaking of Social Welfare*, London: Sage.

Cochrane, A. (1994) 'Managing change in local government', in J. Clarke, A. Cochrane and E. McLaughlin (eds) *Managing Social Policy*, London: Sage.

Craig, G. (1998) 'The privatization of human misery', *Critical Social Policy*, 18, 1: 51–76.

Cutler, T. and Waine, B. (1994) *Managing the Welfare State*, London: Berg.

——(1997) 'The politics of quasi-markets: how quasi-markets have been analysed and how they might be analysed', *Critical Social Policy*, 17, 2: 3–26.

Ferlie, E., Pettigrew, A., Ashburner, L. and Fitzgerald, L. (1996) *The New Public Management in Action*, Oxford: Oxford University Press.

Flynn, N. (1994) 'Control, commitment and contracts', in J. Clarke, A. Cochrane and E. McLaughlin (eds) *Managing Social Policy*, London: Sage.

Green, J. and Armstrong, D. (1995) 'Achieving rational management: bed management and the crisis in emergency admissions', *Sociological Review*, 43, 4: 743–64.

Harrison, S., Hunter, D., Marnoch, J. and Pollitt, C. (1992) *Just Managing: Power and Culture in the National Health Service*, Basingstoke: Macmillan.

Hoggett, P. (1996) 'New modes of control in the public service', *Public Administration*, 74, 9–32.

Huxham, C. (1996) *Creating Collaborative Advantage*, London: Sage.

Kanter, R.M. (1994) 'Collaborative advantage: the art of alliances', *Harvard Business Review*, July–August, 96–108.

Langan, M. (ed.) (1998a) *Welfare: Needs, Rights and Risks: Accessing Social Welfare*, London: Routledge.

——(1998b) 'The restructuring of health care', in G. Hughes and G. Lewis (eds) *Unsettling Welfare*, London: Routledge.

——(1998c) 'Rationing health care', in M. Langan (ed.) *Welfare: Needs, Rights and Risks*, London: Routledge.

Langan, M. and Clarke, J. (1994) 'Managing in the mixed economy of care', in J. Clarke, A. Cochrane and E. McLaughlin (eds) *Managing Social Policy*, London: Sage.

Le Grand, J. and Bartlett, W. (eds) (1993) *Quasi-Markets and Social Policy*, Basingstoke: Macmillan.

Mackintosh, M. (1995) 'Competition and contracting in selective social provision', *European Journal of Development Research*, 7, 1: 26–52.

Mohan, J. (1995) *A National Health Service? The Restructuring of Health Care in Britain since 1979*, Basingstoke: Macmillan.

Nettleton, S. (1996) 'Women and the new paradigm of health and medicine', *Critical Social Policy*, 16, 3: 33–54.

Newman, J. (1998) 'Managerialism and social welfare', in G. Hughes and G. Lewis (eds) *Unsettling Welfare*, London: Routledge.

Pinkney, S. (1998) 'The reshaping of social work and social care', in G. Hughes and G. Lewis (eds) *Unsettling Welfare*, London: Routledge.

Pollitt, C. (1993) *Managerialism and the Public Services*, Oxford: Basil Blackwell (second edition).

Salter, B. (1993) 'The politics of purchasing in the National Health Service', *Policy and Politics*, 21, 3: 171–84.

Stewart, J. (1993) *Accountability to the Public*, London: European Policy Forum.

Twigg, J. (1997) 'Deconstructing the "social bath": help with bathing at home for older and disabled people', *Journal of Social Policy*, 26, 2: 211–32.

Vickridge, R. (1995) 'NHS reforms and community care – means tested health care masquerading as consumer choice?', *Critical Social Policy*, 43, 76–80.

Waldegrave, W. (1993) *The Reality of Reform and Accountability in Today's Public Services*, London: Public Finance Foundation.

Walsh, K. (1995) *Public Services and Market Mechanisms: Competition, Contracting and the New Public Management*, Basingstoke: Macmillan.

Williams, F. (1996) 'Postmodernism, feminism and the question of difference', in N. Parton (ed.) *Social Theory, Social Change and Social Work*, London: Routledge.

4   The health of which nation?

Health, social regulation and the new consensus

Michael Purdy

Introduction

During the 1990s two national health strategies have been developed by British governments for promoting health and reducing rates of preventable illness and premature death in the general population of England. This chapter focuses on these strategies and is concerned with the fact that both *The Health of the Nation* (DOH 1992) and *Our Healthier Nation* (DOH 1998), far from enhancing the health of the whole nation, promote opportunities which are not equitably distributed. Instead, the strategies reinforce the existing 'inverse care law' (Tudor Hart 1971) and generate new divisions and inequalities as 'health' is increasingly regarded as the outcome of informed free choice and as the emblem of the socially responsible citizen, whilst its attainment is denied to those most in need of it. Tied to a technology of individual self-surveillance, those who are either unwilling or unable to be healthy ultimately find themselves excluded from citizenship in the emerging new consensus on welfare.

New Labour

On 5 February 1998, New Labour launched its Green Paper on public health, *Our Healthier Nation* (DOH 1998). Much had been expected of this emerging health strategy. The appointment of a Minister for Public Health and a commitment to advance healthy public policies across all government departments seemed to suggest that the Green Paper would offer an approach to the question of 'the nation's health' radically different from that forwarded in the previous Tory administration's *The Health of the Nation* (DOH 1992).

That a different approach to promoting public health should be demanded of New Labour is indicated by the failure of Tory administrations since 1979 to engage with the 'structural' causes of ill health and premature death. There have been constant calls for central government action to reduce health inequalities by tackling the social and economic conditions which are responsible for them (for example, Townsend and Davidson 1982, Jacobson *et al.* 1991, Whitehead 1992, BMA 1995, Benzeval *et al.* 1995, Wilkinson 1996). These inequalities in morbidity and mortality rates have been shown to exist along many social dimensions in the UK, including those of social class, gender, geographical location, and ethnic background (DOH 1995). Most worrying of all, for more than twenty years commentators have pointed to the alarming fact that the gap between those with the shortest and most disease-ridden lives and those enjoying the longest and healthiest lives has actually been increasing (Brotherston 1976, Phillimore *et al.* 1994, Drever and Whitehead 1997, Richardson and Reid 1997, Acheson 1998, Shaw *et al.* 1998). Since 1979, government policy has marginalised debate in this area, rejecting the recommendations of the Black Report and then attempting to 'bury it' (Timmins 1995), denying any link between poverty and health and restricting Sir Donald Acheson's inquiry into the relative neglect of the public health (DHSS 1988) by failing to ask the committee of inquiry to explore the social factors underlying health.

Against this background, the first indications of New Labour's health strategy are, however, extremely disappointing. Far from offering a structural approach to public health, New Labour appears to want to give us more of the same. What is most striking about *Our Healthier Nation* is its similarity to *The Health of the Nation*, not its difference. Both initiatives present themselves as strategies that aim to enhance and promote the health of the English nation. In point of fact, neither promote equity in health, a goal which has been viewed as central to any health promotion strategy (WHO 1985), but instead generate new divisions and inequalities. In so doing, health promotion strategies such as these are central to the development of new forms of governance and the emergence of a new consensus over welfare.

The health of the nation

The exclusion of those with the poorest health in the UK from healthier and longer lives has been encouraged since 1992 by *The*

Health of the Nation strategy. For the manner in which health was defined and 'targeted', and in particular the effort at apportioning responsibility to individuals themselves for their 'preventable' illnesses and 'premature' deaths, combined to make it increasingly difficult for those with the worst health to experience improvement.

The strategy involved the identification of five key areas for action within each of which specific national objectives and targets are set. The five areas are coronary heart disease and stroke, cancers, mental illness, HIV/AIDS and sexual health, and accidents. Three criteria were employed to select the key areas: 'the area should be a major cause of premature death or avoidable ill-health, effective interventions should be possible, offering significant scope for improvements in health [and] it should be possible to set objectives and targets, and monitor progress towards them' (DOH 1992: 15).

The narrow selection and tight focus on the five areas chosen appears to have been demanded by the need to establish clear priorities, 'so that action and resources can be directed to best effect' (ibid.). By 'best effect' is meant lower cost, insofar as the choice of key areas has been made according to the criteria of both greatest need – a characteristic shared by all of the potential areas due to their status as major killers or disablers – and 'greatest scope for making cost effective improvements' (ibid.). The impact of the drive for cost effectiveness on the strategy is considerable. Indeed, a major attraction of health promotion strategies as compared to health care provision is the belief 'that preventing the onset of illness could reduce health service costs' (Baggott 1994: 243).

A medical model of health

The strategy's focus on key areas which constitute 'major causes of premature death or avoidable ill-health' leads it to endorse a medical model of health as absence of disease/illness. Indeed, the failure of *The Health of the Nation* 'to establish what is meant by health or health promotion' results in its 'distinctly biomedical orientation towards health' (MacDonald 1998: 64). This is necessary because 'the nation's health', and improvements to it brought about through the strategy, have to be measurable, quantifiable and demonstrable. As such, morbidity and mortality rates occupy a central place in the strategy.

A reliance on morbidity and mortality rates makes the identification of 'healthy' and 'unhealthy' behaviours extremely easy. Drinking alcohol, smoking, eating too much saturated fat, getting no exercise, and engaging in irresponsible sexual behaviour are all unhealthy behaviours in that they are linked to preventable illness or premature death. Actively pursuing a wider, positive and more holistic concept of health would make the identification of 'risky' behaviours and unhealthy lifestyles far more problematic. Smoking and drinking alcohol may shorten life and contribute to the development of chronic illness, but this does not necessarily mean that the person, family or community so affected is unhealthy if quality of life is far more important than its length or illness profile. Sex, drugs and rock 'n' roll may shorten your life, but equally they may be pleasurable, high-quality experiences.

Endorsing the medical view of health has significant repercussions. Specifically, it enables two coexisting and mutually available strategies to be activated. On the one hand, a strategy of targeting intrinsically unhealthy behaviours and lifestyles can be pursued – for example, 'excessive' levels of tobacco, saturated fat and alcohol consumption. At the same time, a strategy of exclusion can operate, by which individuals, families, sections of the population, communities and localities which form the support for these behaviours and lifestyles, and in which they are concentrated, can be excluded from the 'healthy nation'. Whilst government via the medical profession defines health, it is individuals, families and communities who are expected to become actively involved in taking responsibility for their own health and ill-health, policing themselves and declaring their membership of 'the nation' through their healthy lifestyles. A central feature of the strategy is therefore the devolving of responsibility for the nation's health to the nation itself. In short, 'health' becomes an active component of citizenship.

This devolving of responsibility for health is expressed through the strategy's emphasis on the role of 'lifestyle choices' and personal behaviour in affecting one's health. The Tory government's message was clear and straightforward, as expressed in its consultative Green Paper (DOH 1991):

> there is considerable emphasis in this document on the need for people to change their behaviour – whether on smoking, alcohol consumption, exercise, diet, avoidance of accidents and, with AIDS, sexual behaviour. The reason is simple. We live in an age where many of these main causes of premature death and unnecessary disease are related to how we live our lives.
>
> (DOH 1991: iv–v)

New Right ideology

The strategy's emphasis on 'lifestyle management' and 'healthy choices' risks divesting both 'lifestyle' and 'choice' of their structural parameters. However, this endorses many features central to Tory 'New Right' thinking, which combines neo-conservative and neo-liberal ideas (Atkinson and Savage 1994).

The neo-liberalist strand focuses on individualist and market-oriented ideas. Here the emphasis is on the absolute primacy of the individual and on protecting the fundamental values of freedom and liberty. Such protection requires an unrestricted free market, which will guarantee freedom by being based on individual choice, and a minimal state whose actions are made compatible with the free market by being limited to the creation of the conditions which enable individuals to exercise freedom of choice, namely the 'rule of law' (Hayek 1944).

The neo-conservative strand, on the other hand, emphasises 'social authoritarian' ideas. Here the concern is with challenges to traditional values and institutions, such as the family, which are seen to have accompanied the increasing 'permissiveness' of modern societies. Unlike neo-liberals, who view the 'state' of contemporary society as the consequence of too little individual freedom in the face of too much state interference, neo-conservatives regard the 'problems' of post-war society as stemming from too much individual freedom, which has resulted in, for example, a breakdown in law and order and a general decline of morality. The focus for neo-conservatives is on the restoration of authority, stability, order and morality. In this, and 'unlike the neo-liberals', 'they place a considerable emphasis upon collectivities and the responsibilities and duties of the individual towards the collectivity' (Atkinson and Savage 1994: 7).

In *The Health of the Nation* it is neo-liberal rather than neo-conservative priorities which dominate. Thus, support for the medicalisation of the strategy is generated by both the new Right ideological agenda of maximising individual responsibility and choice, and by the political need to demonstrate the effectiveness of health promotion strategies in reducing the financial burden of an increasingly expensive health care system. Medical discourse is employed to define the health promotion objectives of the national strategy by limiting these objectives to quantifiable (and therefore achievable) reductions in the incidence of disease and death in key areas which appear open to the successful utilisation of the medical model with its emphasis on the impact of individual lifestyle choices on disease causation and premature death.

New Right assumptions concerning individuals' freedom to choose are clearly confirmed by a health strategy in which an emphasis on lifestyle management dominates. Thus, in the Green Paper, 'the need to address social inequalities' is absent (Radical Statistics Health Group 1991), and the strategy 'never considers making social inequalities in health a key area' (Delamothe 1991). Instead, the cornerstone of government action on health is seen to be to facilitate 'informed free choice' (DOH 1991: v), and in the subsequent White Paper there is a clear endorsement of the assumption that individuals choose their lifestyle (DOH 1992: 11).

Our healthier nation

Whilst an emphasis on the personal management of lifestyle endorses elements of New Right thinking, it is not confined to this ideological tradition. For the 'high risk' approach to health promotion and the prevention of disease found in *The Health of the Nation*, in which the 'unhealthy' lifestyles of those groups most at risk from 'lifestyle diseases' are targeted, has a long cross-party pedigree. In 1976 the Labour government published *Prevention and Health: Everybody's Business* (DHSS 1976), in which individual lifestyle is held to be responsible for many health problems, and in 1987 the White Paper *Promoting Better Health* (DOH 1987) argued that if people took more responsibility for their health, major killer diseases could be avoided. In 1998 we find New Labour again targeting the lifestyles and choices of those experiencing the poorest health in its consultative Green Paper *Our Healthier Nation* (DOH 1998).

What distinguishes the new strategy from that of *Health of the Nation*, according to the government, is its acknowledgement of 'the social, economic and environmental causes of ill health' (DOH 1998: 57), an acknowledgement which includes the explicit recognition of the link between poverty and ill health. Consequently the new strategy will seek to tackle these conditions by adopting what the government refers to as a 'third way', which avoids both 'individual victim blaming' and 'nanny state social engineering' (ibid.: 28). Instead, New Labour is proposing a 'contract for health' which recognises that the causes of ill health are not government's or individual's alone but rather shared by society and therefore require a partnership between government, communities and individuals to achieve the strategy's two key aims, which are:

To improve the health of the population as a whole by increasing the length of people's lives and the number of years people spend free from illness.

To improve the health of the worst off in society and to narrow the health gap.

(ibid.: 5)

Central to government's role in this partnership will be to act on 'the things' beyond individuals' control which damage health and lead to fundamental inequalities, such as air pollution, poverty, low wages, unemployment, poor housing and crime. Local organisations and agencies are charged with taking the lead in operationalising the strategy insofar as: 'Whilst Government can set a framework...it is people on the ground, working locally and directly with communities, who can do most to make *Our Healthier Nation* a reality' (ibid.: 39). And finally, individuals have a role, which is 'to choose whether to change their behaviour to a healthier one' (ibid.: 48).

Despite its desire to 'narrow the health gap', the New Labour strategy is remarkably similar to its Tory predecessor in refusing to target inequalities in health as a key national priority and in delegating responsibility for reducing such inequalities to local initiatives. In New Labour's case the key mechanisms for tackling inequalities in health are identified as the local 'health improvement programmes', which its structural changes to the NHS will set in motion (DOH 1997a), its piloting of Health Action Zones (DOH 1997b), and the establishing of a network of Healthy Living Centres (DSS 1998, DOH 1999).

Whilst the government does not rule out the possibility of considering 'the scope for national targets on inequalities' (DOH 1998: 83, Crail 1998), it is clear that its preference is to set few national targets, thereby 'offering greater flexibility to focus on particular local health problems' (DOH 1998: 80). In fact, the government proposes to reduce the number considerably from that of *The Health of the Nation*, setting only one target in each of four priority areas. The priority areas are identical to four of the five key areas established by the Tory strategy, namely heart disease and stroke, accidents, cancer, and mental health.

The government's wish to increase the scope for local flexibility by cutting the number of national targets nevertheless obscures a fundamental tension between local autonomy and central authority. For, just as in the Tory strategy, local action on health is to be closely monitored. Thus, in its restructuring of the NHS (DOH 1997a), New Labour establishes mechanisms of central, regional and local policing of the implementation of centrally agreed local 'health improvement programmes'.

Through its choice of national targets New Labour retains the medical model of health which characterised *The Health of the Nation*, along with the strategies of targeting unhealthy behaviours and of excluding the unhealthy from the nation which medicalisation permits.

In targeting unhealthy behaviours the government is careful to distance itself from the 'victim blaming' which has come to be associated with the earlier Tory strategy. As it states: 'Good health is no longer about blame, but about opportunity and responsibility' (DOH 1998: 5). Here New Labour signals its view that health is a 'social responsibility' of the individual, arguing that, whilst the individual cannot be forced to choose a healthier lifestyle, it is important for us all to be aware of our responsibilities towards those around us in the lifestyle choices that we make. Specifically, the government emphasises the fundamental importance of the family unit and of parents in providing role models for the health-related behaviour of the young:

> Individual responsibility is not only about our own health. It is also about the example that we set to those around us. The example and boundaries that parents set are central to the health of their children. It is in stable and caring families that children learn the self-confidence to become secure and independent individuals.
>
> (ibid.: 48)

In emphasising that the 'healthy choice' is the 'socially responsible' choice, New Labour echoes and endorses the neo-conservative theme of the individual's responsibility to society. Moreover, emphasising one's social responsibility to be healthy does not sever links with 'victim blaming' as cleanly as the government would wish.

Healthy lifestyles

New Labour's focus on 'lifestyle management' may be conducted in a discourse that is less abrasive than that of the Tory New Right, but it nonetheless emphasises the desirability for individuals to adjust their lifestyles. As such, the strategy is liable both to exclude those who need public health measures the most and to lead to 'healthism', in which the unhealthy run the risk of becoming increasingly marginalised.

Excluding the unhealthy

That health strategies which call on people to adjust their lifestyles should disadvantage those with the poorest health and greatest need is due to the fact that the individuals, families and communities who suffer the most ill health lack opportunities to effect the healthy choices called for. They may 'have little or no spare capacity and few or no resources to make the necessary changes' (Francome and Marks 1996: 272). Moreover, an emphasis on individual behavioural change may actually increase inequalities in health, insofar as the personal gains to be made from following health educational advice become available to those who need them least (Adams 1994, Nettleton and Bunton 1995). As Leichter puts it: 'It may well be that wellness...is being wasted on the well' (1997: 375). So, if the concentration of preventable illness and premature death in particular sections of the UK population (DOH 1995) is taken into account, then the 'lifestyle approach' of health promotion strategies places the responsibility for ill health squarely on the shoulders of those who suffer most. Health promotion strategies may therefore both confirm and extend the 'inverse care law' (Tudor Hart 1971, Benzeval and Judge 1996).

The inadequacy of this approach lies in the ease with which the significance of structural features that enable choices to be made is either forgotten or rendered invisible. New Labour's emphasis on the key role of the family in delivering health to its members, for instance, appears to ignore material constraints, which can mean: 'The freedom of each family to choose its own lifestyle is more illusion than reality' (Cresson and Pitrou 1991: 215).

Characteristically, health promotion strategies view choice as the outcome of a process of rational deliberation and calculation undertaken by informed individuals, whose knowledge of health risks enables them to adjust their lifestyle in order to protect their health. Any limitations or barriers to those suffering the poorest health making such choices are regarded as the result of ignorance. The assumption is that the provision of information on the risks to health of certain behaviours and lifestyles 'empowers' a population to make the 'healthy choice'.

The logic of the health education imperative found in health promotion strategies is seriously flawed, and its view of free choice highly problematic. For it fails to acknowledge both the importance of the social, cultural and economic contexts within which individuals and families make their decisions and act, and the rationality of the 'choices' which they make.

Both Hilary Graham and Clare Blackburn have drawn attention to the rationalities that structure and inform the apparently unhealthy behaviour of those experiencing some of the poorest health in our country. Blackburn (1991), for example, demonstrates that unhealthy food choices, which are so often attributed to the 'ignorance and irresponsible behaviour' of those that make them, are in fact related to material and social factors such as low income and available shopping facilities. Indeed, far from being irresponsible and irrational in their food choices, 'Low-income families shop more efficiently in money and nutritional terms than higher income families' (1991: 55).

In her work on smoking behaviour amongst low-income women, Graham (1993, 1996) similarly reveals the presence of rationalities at work in behaviour which is so often and so casually written off as illogical, irrational and irresponsible. Here smoking is undertaken in the full knowledge of its health-damaging effects to both smoker and others for the assistance it gives the women in caring for their families in situations characterised by inadequate material resources and high levels of stress and anxiety. In such circumstances, unhealthy smoking behaviour has to be understood in the context of these women's everyday lives, a context of 'Caring for more and living on less' (1993: 98) in which this unhealthy behaviour appears less as a poor 'choice' than as a rational 'compromise':

> Cigarette smoking was experienced as a child-protective strategy, a resource which helped mothers cope with the demands of caring, both on a routine basis and through the periods of stress and crisis that punctuated their lives. For the mothers in this study, habits like smoking were experienced less as a lifestyle choice and more as a life compromise, taken, in the full knowledge of the health risks, to protect the welfare of the family.
>
> (1996: 176)

Smoking is not, therefore, simply a matter of individual choice of lifestyle. Rather, it reproduces through its prevalence and distribution economic differences in 'life chances'. As such: 'Poverty and economic inequality – not smoking – could...be argued to be the most important health hazard in late-twentieth century Britain' (Pond and Popay 1993: 185).

Healthism

Healthism has been defined as

> the preoccupation with personal health as a primary – often *the* primary – focus for the definition and achievement of well-being; a goal which is to be attained primarily through the modification of life styles.
>
> (Crawford 1980: 368)

The focus on personal health and on individual management of lifestyle diverts attention from the social basis of disease and ill health, sustaining an ideology of 'victim blaming' (Crawford 1977) in which individuals appear to be responsible for their own health. The World Health Organisation (WHO) attempts to distance itself from 'healthism' (WHO 1986), warning against imposing healthy lifestyles on people, the essence of health promotion being 'choice'. People must therefore be free to refuse 'healthy choices', however: 'at the same time people should assume their social responsibilities towards each other' (ibid.: 123). The dangers to which the forging of links between healthy choices and social responsibility can lead should not be underestimated. Victim blaming may be avoided in recognising, as WHO does, limitations on freedom of choice, but avoidance, rejection or failure to *access* health (promotion) strategies can also be read as acts of social deviancy, in which: 'Failure to act preventively becomes a sign of a *social*, not just individual, irresponsibility' (Crawford 1980: 379).

In the case of New Labour, recognition that, for some groups in the United Kingdom, the opportunities for 'choosing' a healthier lifestyle are severely limited by 'social and economic factors' such as poverty, unemployment and social exclusion (DOH 1998: 16–17), leads to a 'partnership' approach in which there is an expectation that if government does its bit to make healthier choices easier for more of the nation, by acting on the 'things' over which individuals have no control, then individuals *should* do the socially responsible thing and make the healthy choice.

In effect, health promotion strategies such as *The Health of the Nation* and *Our Healthier Nation* construct health in such a way as to exclude sections of the population from 'the nation', sections that for one reason or another cannot or will not endorse through their behaviour a norm of 'healthy living'. The risk here is that different and minority lifestyles that do not fit cleanly into the 'healthy norm' may become regarded as deviant, undesirable and even dangerous. Moreover, the privileging of health as a cultural norm and its equating with rational behaviour denies the cultural validity of alternative discourses to that of health promotion. As Thorogood observes:

> Here then is an inherent tension for health promotion. To acknowledge the possibility of choice within discourses other than health as equally valid would undermine health promotion's claim to scientific rationality. If health promotion were truly to accept all choices as equally valid, the role of *health* promotion would be reduced to promoting access to and decision making about services, and the dominance of the rational, medico-scientific paradigm would be challenged. It would be possible for other social formations to arise, for competing social norms and values to move into ascendance.
>
> (1992: 61)

Health and social regulation

Thorogood's observation points to the intimate link between health promotion and 'social regulation' and to the fact that 'In contemporary western societies the concept of health has become central to the construction of subjectivities' (Lupton 1995: 69). This regulatory function of health promotion and of the new public health strategies operates not so much by explicitly challenging and rejecting particular lifestyles and the individuals and communities that support them as by encouraging and endorsing specific attitudes towards health and associated practices of 'self-regulation'. In short, health promotion introduces 'new forms of social regulation which are not ostensibly oppressive nor obviously controlling' (Bunton 1992: 10).

Central to the establishing of a norm of health and of healthy living is a discourse of 'risk'. This discourse suggests that contemporary society is a society saturated by risk, in which the health of all is potentially threatened (Petersen 1997). Risk is therefore 'individualised' insofar as everyone is a potential target. To guard against the threat, individuals must be vigilant, take responsibility for their lives and manage themselves by 'regulating the self' through continual risk-surveillance. Health promotion and the new public health therefore operate principally by producing 'healthy subjectivities' rather than by constraining or condemning unhealthy ones. The threat of external sanctions or 'punishment' of unhealthy behaviour is rarely necessary. Instead, the socially responsible citizen monitors his or her behaviour and lifestyle for contamination by unhealthy foods, drinks, drugs and pastimes, which can then be purged through the exercise of individual (healthy) choices. In this respect, health promotion and the new public health strategies exist as significant discourses enabling individuals to govern themselves.

An increasing emphasis upon 'governing the self' is present in the new consensus on welfare that is gradually emerging in the wake of the restructuring of state welfarism experienced in the 1980s and 1990s. For this new consensus relies on a principle of 'respon-sibilisation' (Osborne 1997), according to which the individual's social *responsibilities* rather than their social *rights* form the basis of citizenship. As such, health ceases to be regarded as a right of citizenship, guaranteed by a welfare state, and instead takes on the appearance of a 'duty of citizenship'. In this new consensus little room will exist for those who fail to govern themselves according to the 'imperative of health'. They will effectively exclude them-selves from the 'healthy nation' through their inability or unwilling-ness to be healthy. Such exclusion testifies to the intolerance of difference which characterises the new consensus and its 'idealisation of the "normal", "healthy" subject' (Petersen and Lupton 1996), an intolerance which sees in 'unhealthiness' nothing but moral failure.

Both *The Health of the Nation* and *Our Healthier Nation* stand as complementary strategies within the space of this emerging new consensus. As strategies that advocate 'lifestyle management' as a solution to ill health and premature death, they are shamefully responsible for compounding existing health inequalities and generating new divisions. The promotion of such inequality clearly sits comfortably with the 'competitive individualism' of Tory New Right ideology. For central to this political process was the creation of 'a system of values which accepts greater inequality as both inevitable and desirable' (Johnson 1990). Unfortunately, New Labour's 'third way' – in which 'Collective rights were to be replaced by individual obligations' (Higgs 1998: 191) – is no less effective in making a new consensus on welfare acceptable to a society which previously and publicly pursued collectivist policies of social justice for more than thirty years. Rather than mimic the Tory strategy, Labour's new public health should start by rediscovering, reactivating and rigorously pursuing those collectivist policies and the values that informed them.

References

Acheson, D. (chair) (1998) *Independent Inquiry into Inequalities in Health Report*, London: The Stationery Office.

Adams, L. (1994) 'Health promotion in crisis', *Health Education Journal* 53, 354–60.

Atkinson, R. and Savage, S. (1994) 'The conservatives and public policy', in S. Savage, R. Atkinson and L. Robins (eds) *Public Policy in Britain*, London: St Martin's Press.

Baggott, B. (1994) *Health and Health Care in Britain*, London: Macmillan.

Benzeval, M. and Judge, K. (1996) 'Access to health care in England: continuing inequalities in the distribution of GPs', *Journal of Public Health Medicine* 18, 1: 33–40.

Benzeval, M., Judge, K. and Whitehead, M. (eds) (1995) *Tackling Inequalities in Health: An Agenda for Action*, London: King's Fund.

Blackburn, C. (1991) *Poverty and Health: Working with Families*, Milton Keynes: Open University Press.

British Medical Association (BMA) (1995) *Inequalities in Health*, London: British Medical Association Board of Science and Education.

Brotherston, J. (1976) 'Inequality: is it inevitable?', in C.O. Carter and J. Peel (eds) *Equalities and Inequalities in Health*, London: Academic Press.

Bunton, R. (1992) 'More than a woolly jumper: health promotion as social regulation', *Critical Public Health* 3, 2: 4–11.

Crail, M. (1998) 'The unequal struggle', *Health Service Journal* 108, 5597: 12–13.

Crawford, R. (1977) 'You are dangerous to your health: the ideology and politics of victim blaming', *International Journal of Health Services* 7, 4: 663–80.

——(1980) 'Healthism and the medicalization of everyday life', *International Journal of Health Services* 10, 3: 365–88.

Cresson, G. and Pitrou, A. (1991) 'The role of the family in creating and maintaining healthy lifestyles', in B. Bandura and I. Kickbusch (eds) *Health Promotion Research: Towards a New Social Epidemiology*, WHO Regional Publications, European Series, No. 37, Copenhagen: WHO Regional Office for Europe.

Delamothe, T. (1991) 'Social inequalities in health', *British Medical Journal* 303, 1046–50.

Department of Health (DOH) (1987) *Promoting Better Health*, London: HMSO.

——(1991) *The Health of the Nation: A Consultative Document for Health in England*, London: HMSO.

——(1992) *The Health of the Nation: A Strategy for Health in England*, London: HMSO.

——(1995) *The Health of the Nation: Variations in Health. What can the Department of Health and the NHS Do?*, Report of the Variations

Sub-Group of the Chief Medical Officer's Health of the Nation Working Group, London: DOH.

——(1997a) *The New NHS: Modern, Dependable*, London: The Stationery Office.

——(1997b) *Health Action Zone: Invitation to Bid*, London: DOH.

——(1998) *Our Healthier Nation: A Contract for Health*, London: The Stationery Office.

——(1999) *Healthy Living Centres*, HSC 1999/008, London: DOH.

Department of Health and Social Security (DHSS) (1976) *Prevention and Health: Everybody's Business*, London: HMSO.

——(1988) *Public Health in England: The Report of the Committee of Inquiry into the Future Development of the Public Health Function*, London: HMSO.

Department of Social Security (DSS) (1998) *New Ambitions for Our Country: A New Contract for Welfare*, London: The Stationery Office.

Drever, F. and Whitehead, M. (eds) (1997) *Health Inequalities*, Office for National Statistics, London: The Stationery Office.

Francome, C. and Marks, D. (1996) *Improving the Health of the Nation: The Failure of the Government's Health Reforms*, London: Middlesex University Press.

Graham, H. (1993) *When Life's a Drag: Women, Smoking and Disadvantage*, London: Department of Health, HMSO.

——(1996) 'Researching women's health work: a study of the lifestyles of women on income support', in P. Bywaters and E. McLeod (eds) *Working for Equality in Health*, London: Routledge.

Hayek, F. (1944) *The Road to Serfdom*, London: Routledge & Kegan Paul.

Higgs, P. (1998) 'Risk, governmentality and the reconceptualisation of citizenship', in G. Scambler and P. Higgs (eds) *Modernity, Medicine and Health*, London: Routledge.

Jacobson, B., Smith, A. and Whitehead, M. (eds) (1991) *The Nation's Health: A Strategy for the 1990s*, report from an Independent Multidisciplinary Committee, revised edition, London: King's Fund.

Johnson, N. (1990) *Reconstructing the Welfare State: A Decade of Change 1980–1990*, London: Harvester Wheatsheaf.

Leichter, H. (1997) 'Lifestyle correctness and the new secular morality', in A. Brandt and P. Rozin (eds) *Morality and Health*, New York: Routledge.

Lupton, D. (1995) *The Imperative of Health: Public Health and the Regulated Body*, London: Sage.

MacDonald, T.H. (1998) *Rethinking Health Promotion: A Global Approach*, London: Routledge.

Nettleton, S. and Bunton, R. (1995) 'Sociological critiques of health promotion', in R. Bunton, S. Nettleton and R. Burrows (eds) *The Sociology of Health Promotion: Critical Analyses of Consumption, Lifestyle and Risk*, London: Routledge.

Osborne, T. (1997) 'Of health and statecraft', in A. Petersen and R. Bunton (eds) *Foucault, Health and Medicine*, London: Routledge.

Petersen, A. (1997) 'Risk, governance and the new public health', in A. Petersen and R. Bunton (eds) *Foucault, Health and Medicine*, London: Routledge.

Petersen, A. and Lupton, D. (1996) *The New Public Health: Health and Self in the Age of Risk*, London: Sage.

Phillimore, P., Beattie, A. and Townsend, P. (1994) 'Widening inequality of health in northern England, 1981–91', *British Medical Journal* 308, 1125–8.

Pond, C. and Popay, J. (1993) 'Poverty, economic inequality and health', in B. Davey and J. Popay (eds) *Dilemmas in Health Care*, Buckingham: Open University Press.

Radical Statistics Health Group (1991) 'Missing: a strategy for health of the nation', *British Medical Journal* 303, 299–302.

Richardson, A. and Reid, G. (1997) *Sheffield and Electoral Ward Mortality Trends, 1981 to 1996*, Sheffield: Sheffield Health, Department of Information and Research.

Shaw, M., Dorling, D. and Brimblecombe, N. (1998) 'Changing the map: health in Britain 1951–1991', *Sociology of Health & Illness* 20, 5: 694–709.

Thorogood, N. (1992) 'What is the relevance of sociology for health promotion?', in R. Bunton and G. Macdonald (eds) *Health Promotion: Disciplines and Diversity*, London: Routledge.

Timmins, N. (1995) *The Five Giants: A Biography of the Welfare State*, London: Fontana Press.

Townsend, P. and Davidson, N. (eds) (1982) 'The Black Report', in P. Townsend, M. Whitehead and N. Davidson (eds) *Inequalities in Health: The Black Report and the Health Divide*, London: Penguin Books.

Tudor Hart, J. (1971) 'The inverse care law', *The Lancet* 27 February: 405–12.

Whitehead, M. (1992) 'The health divide', in P. Townsend, M. Whitehead and N. Davidson (eds) *Inequalities in Health: The Black Report and the Health Divide*, London: Penguin Books.

Wilkinson, R. (1996) *Unhealthy Societies: From Inequality to Well-Being*, London: Routledge.

World Health Organisation (WHO) (1985) *Targets for Health for All: Targets in Support of the European Regional Strategy for Health for All*, Copenhagen: WHO Regional Office for Europe.

——(1986) 'Lifestyles and health', *Social Science and Medicine* 22, 2: 117–24.

5 Exclusion in maternity care
Midwives and mothers

Mavis Kirkham

Introduction

The anthropologist Brigitte Jordan states that:

> In order to deal with [the] danger and the existential uncertainty associated with birth, people tend to produce a set of internally consistent and mutually dependent practices and beliefs that are designed to manage the physiologically and socially problematic aspects of parturition in a way that makes sense in that particular cultural context. It is not surprising, therefore, that – whatever the details of a given birthing system – its practitioners will tend to see it as the best way, the right way, indeed *the* way to bring a child into the world.
>
> (Jordan 1983: 4)

With cultural change and different social powerholders, the definitions of the right way to give birth have changed. The power of the church, the professions and the market have marked the experience of childbearing women and their carers over succeeding centuries. This chapter aims to outline the move from women supporting childbearing friends and witnessing birth, to the professional control and management of childbearing. This process demonstrates, in the earlier period, the exclusion of women as primary carers, and, more recently, exclusion by women as subordinate carers.

Since 'the problematic aspects of parturition' (Jordan 1983, quoted above) are managed in a way that 'makes sense' within the values of social powerholders, the 'right way' to conduct birth is difficult to question. The voice of those less socially powerful is muted, even though they give birth and deliver the babies, and their dependence upon those who control the 'right way' to give birth is considerable. Those who are excluded from independent clinical practice or from receiving maternity care appropriate to their needs, still continue to provide care and to give birth. Issues of exclusion and dependency are therefore intertwined and mutually sustaining.

For the purpose of this chapter, a midwife is defined as one (almost always female) who gives care around childbirth, during labour and who receives the baby at delivery. The word midwife means 'with woman', and the midwife, or grace-wife as she was known in some areas (Wilson 1995), supported the childbearing woman who was the active partner in the birth. Traditionally there are many examples of midwives' skills in surgery and medicine, and the current international definition (WHO 1965) fits into modern medical practice. Nevertheless, the key characteristic in definitions of the work of the midwife is her care and support around, rather than intervention in, the process of childbearing.

The exclusion of midwives from independent clinical practice

The pre-industrial period

Care of women in labour and birth was traditionally women's work in this country. Whilst midwifery was part of a wider female healing role, birth was definitely 'women's business'. 'Lying-ins were thus exempt from the male control that extended over almost all other aspects of a woman's life' (Blumenfeld-Kosinski 1990). Birth, its many rituals and the midwives and 'gossips' involved in each birth, can be seen as the pivot of a female culture which, though socially limited, played a key part in the lives of women of all social classes.

There were inevitably tensions about the control of midwifery. The midwife presided over a child's entrance to society, was responsible for the soul of any baby unlikely to survive until a church baptism, and was closely involved with the health and fertility of the mother. In all these areas she could be seen as challenging the control of male powerholders. A midwife who inspires self-confidence in childbearing women has a powerful skill, and the potential challenge of this skill was answered with control or condemnation as witchcraft. While ordinances, therefore, ensured that 'good' midwives were controlled, first by the church and later by the state via the medical profession, 'bad' midwives were uncontrolled and perceived as threatening to the social order. 'It is clear how professionalisation and witchcraft intersect: both achieving similar ends with regard to society as a whole and to the healing professions in particular: they marginalised women' (Blumenfeld-Kosinski 1990: 110).

The 1512 Act, which made the first formal arrangements for the control of midwives in England, strengthened the control of the church. Midwives were required to swear before the Bishop's Court to 'faithfully and diligently exercise the office' of midwife and to use no 'sorcery or incantations'. As the priest had no access to the women's world of birth, midwives were required to produce 'six honest matrons' whom they had delivered during their period of instruction who would testify to their skill (Donnison 1977). Thus the first Act to license and control midwives in England emphasised their mutual dependence with the women of their community.

In many European cities, midwives became salaried by the munici-palities and thus gained a new and financially secure status whilst providing a free service within their city. This progress was achieved by a process of control. 'The independent and competent women practitioners of the early Middle Ages are replaced, in the latter Middle Ages, by women caught up in a web of medical regulations and municipal ordinances' (Blumenfeld-Kosinski 1990: 91). The degree of control varied, but could not be total until men had entrance to the birth chamber.

Until around 1720, the role of the male 'surgeon' in childbirth was very largely confined to obstructed labours, where he was called to dismember and extricate the dead foetus with hooks, in order to save the life of the mother. Thus women dreaded calling a male practi-tioner, for all that symbolised of death and destruction. Whilst obstetric forceps (first used in the seventeenth century) have been described as 'the key to the lying-in room' (Radcliffe 1967), entrance was only achieved after profound cultural change. Understanding the process of this change 'has been hampered by male scholarly bias in the historiography of medicine as well as that of witchcraft' (Blumenfeld-Kosinski 1990). Many midwives were illiterate, and key texts in the history of childbirth were often written by those who were competing with them for trade. Thus accounts of midwives' practice tended to create a picture of 'meddlesome' women with very limited skill, who, at their very best, were 'nature's servants' (Willughby 1972), and to imply that this had always been the case.

In this context earlier, post-mortem caesarean sections are impor-tant because those who carried them out intervened in a natural process and exercised several socially important skills: the diagnosis of maternal death and the use of surgical instruments to ensure a rapid delivery of a child whose soul was then saved by baptism. Caesarean birth is also revealing because it has been portrayed in art for many centuries, whereas the illustration of normal birth would have been seen as immodest until relatively recently. Blumenfeld-Kosinski's study of medical texts and of art concerning post-mortem caesarean birth documented a change, from female to male attendants: 'The fourteenth century midwives, acting so competently and energetically, have no place in the fifteenth century' (1990: 90). Thus the change was social, alongside very early moves to professionalise medicine and long before there were any issues of skill or equipment in terms of saving maternal life.

For several centuries midwives continued to care for childbearing neighbours as part of the fabric of their domestic life. Men and women cooperated in maintaining a social order whereby:

> It was the ceremony of childbirth that conferred authority on the midwife; the woman's personal choice only extended to *which* midwife...would deliver her. What gave the ritual its immense power was collective female authority...Mothers, midwives and gossips were bound together by the same web of social bonds that constituted the collective culture of women in general. That culture was made possible by the range of experiences and activities shared by mothers of all social ranks. The basis of this sharing was the patriarchal order...Even the aristocratic wife was subsumed within that order; all women were bound by it. Hence the fact that the relatively humble midwife could assert power over a mother who belonged to the ruling class.
>
> (Wilson 1995: 185)

This 'collective culture of women' started to fragment in the seventeenth century. Wilson saw this as largely due to the advent of literacy and leisure for women of the upper classes. A culture of ladies developed 'distinct from that of their husbands and from that of humbler women' (ibid.: 187). Thus ladies gained a degree of independence which was real, though defined in male terms. The midwife, 'by her very presence...served as a tangible reminder that ladies were merely women'. As the practice of male midwives came, through the use of the vectis and forceps, to be associated with the birth of live children, they also offered clients 'proof of their superior social status: who but ladies could afford the 10 guineas that William Hunter charged for deliveries?' (ibid.: 191). 'Fashion was the symbolic reflection of the new culture of class...the artisan's wife might not be able to afford a carriage, but every couple of years she could afford a man-midwife. Man-midwifery thus became an area of conspicuous consumption' (ibid.). This shift was aided by the considerable efforts of male practitioners to ally with some aspects of the female culture of birth. 'William Hunter, in delineating the route to male practice as a midwife, laid great stress upon pleasing and appeasing the "gossips" and never mentioned husbands in this connection.'

The economic changes which made leisure possible for ladies were built upon a firm delineation between domestic and occupational roles. The shift in the dominant location of medical services from the private domestic to the public market arena 'sounded the death knell for women's medical practice' (Witz 1992: 82).

The nineteenth century

The troubled relations between midwives and medical men can be seen as 'a paradigmatic case of gendered demarcationary strategies in the emerging medical division of labour' (Witz 1992: 104). Medical men engaged in 'a demarcation strategy of de-skilling' around the definition of normal childbirth (the midwife's area of practice) and abnormal childbirth (the medical area). They also sought to 'ossify this division of labour' by containing and controlling the practice of normal midwifery. The midwives involved in the protracted debates about midwifery registration were very different from those of earlier centuries. Historical studies show that the higher status of professions within the occupational structure does not rest on technical skills alone, but is supported by their members' origins in 'groups already enjoying high status and power in society' (Elliot 1972). Such status was never held by the average midwife, who was poor, often illiterate and working irregularly. The Midwives Institute, however, represented 'not the whole of midwifery, but the views and interests of the elite leadership' (Heagerty 1990).

Celia Davis has argued that a profession's ideology and strategy come not from a consensus amongst its members but 'the "official" view as propounded by leaders' (Davis 1983). Those leading the campaign for higher training and status for midwifery, and therefore for state registration, were Victorian ladies. They were members of the upper classes created by industry and trade who were consigned to leisure because they were female, but, sharing the reforming zeal of many of their class, they sought opportunities to improve the lot of others through occupations suitable for ladies. The professionalisation of midwifery was thus an ideal project; a traditional female role could be raised to a social level from which ladies could improve the lot of childbearing women. Being female, the ladies of the Midwives Institute did not have access to the resources necessary to achieve their aims. They therefore worked by proxy through sympathetic men of their social class, which included many great social reformers. They did this with a skill highly developed in reforming Victorian ladies and not unknown in midwives today.

Achieving the 1902 Midwives Act

In the debates which preceded the 1902 Act, there were three ways in which different interests approached the issue of care around childbirth with vastly different implications for midwives.

1   To secure highly skilled midwives who would effectively be specialised medical practitioners. The women's organisations which took this position were seen as too challenging to win powerful allies.
2   To dissolve the independent midwifery role into that of an obstetric or monthly nurse who 'under the charge and supervision of a medical man, carries out that portion of attendance which is more suitable to a mere woman, the changing of sheets and attending to the patient, and attentions of that kind' (HMSO 1892: 133). This option was much supported by GPs and was what prevailed in the USA.
3   To preserve the role of the midwife as an independent practitioner within the strictly defined sphere of normal childbearing. Such a role admitted the superior status of doctors but relieved them of 'tiring and unremunerative work' (ibid.: 22). This fitted the world view of many of the aristocrats of British medicine, who saw midwifery as 'an occupation degrading to a gentleman' (Smith 1979: 23).

This third view, which was to prevail in 1902, assured both the continuance of midwifery and its control by medical men. This Act enshrined the education of midwives in law and ensured that this education, 'kept necessarily and designedly limited' (HMSO 1892: 112), kept them in their place. 'What you want to educate midwives for is for them to know their own ignorance. That is really the one great object in educating midwives' (ibid.: 101). This was a far cry from the earlier situation where 'the midwife was the women's doctor...of early modern England' (Wilson 1995: 38).

The professionalisation of midwifery: ladies and women

At a time when 'in the context of late nineteenth-century medical care delivery, lay midwives offered at least as safe a service to parturient women as physicians' (Heagerty 1990), the campaigners for midwifery's future were a very different group. They were the spinsters of a social class whose childbearing women were no longer attended by midwives. The Midwives Institute's early members trained in the most prestigious midwifery courses then rapidly became leaders of maternity and philanthropic institutions, as befitted their position in society. The midwife members of the Institute's Council were all trained nurses and thus deferred to male medical authority.

At a time when even privileged women suffered from social and political inequality, the Institute offered a haven where they could gain mutual support and work for a high ideal. Beyond making mandatory the registration and training of midwives, they sought to improve the quality of midwifery attendance for the working class and at the same time to reform working-class habits and values. The midwife must aim 'to exert a wholesome influence over her patients...to raise and refine their feelings and make them see the benefit of cleanliness and order' (*Nursing Notes*, March 1890). They worked for this with a missionary zeal that was grounded in their social class. The professional elite sought formal training for midwives partly to change the tone of midwifery by changing its social class structure (Heagerty 1990).

From this viewpoint, the 1902 Midwives Act was only a partial victory as it allowed lay midwives to register and continue to practise as 'bona fide' midwives. The key argument against bona fide midwives – that their practice put childbearing women at increased risk of infection – was not substantiated. One Inspector of Midwives surveyed her 1907–1918 statistics and found, 'The figures show the lowest death rate amongst mothers attended by the very women that the Midwives Act 1902 was passed to do away with' (*Nursing Notes*, March 1931). Nevertheless, the Central Midwives Board and Local Supervising Authorities showed little understanding of the realities of these midwives' lives:

> the midwife herself was expected to conform to the moral and cultural standards of middle-class social reformers, rather than those of the working-class community in which most midwives had their roots. From this framework of stipulations and restric-

tions would emerge the ideal midwife: one who no longer placed the women she attended before her submission to the medical profession and her deference to her social betters.

(Heagarty 1990: 82)

This fundamental shift in allegiance lay at the heart of the professionalisation of midwifery. The basic contradiction contained within the term 'professional midwife', with the very different primary allegiances implied in those two words, demonstrates the tensions within midwifery then and very recently. Inevitably, the professionalisation process embarked upon by the ladies of the Midwives Institute could only produce a 'subordinate profession' or 'semi-profession' (Etzioni 1969) suited to the role of 'handmaidens of a male occupation that had authority over them' (Simpson and Simpson 1969).

Professional aspirations and expectations necessitated the exclusion of the working-class midwife, grounded in her community, from professional practice. Rank and file midwives supported, and were supported by, the women of their community, as shown in the petitions in support of many midwives subject to disciplinary processes. From the other side of an unbridgeable social divide, midwifery reformers continued to place responsibility for the country's high infant and maternal mortality with 'ignorant working-class mothers and untrained midwives'. The Department of Health attributed blame similarly (Campbell 1924). Yet bona fide midwives continued to support mothers, not just during labour but by helping them with domestic work after the delivery. Qualified midwives were not willing to perform these menial but vital tasks, 'as well as being more expensive, they were of less use to women' (Isherwood 1992). Nevertheless, the bona fide midwives' social position meant that they lacked a political voice. Around 1910 a midwives trades union was formed, but it disappeared during World War I. From then on the voice of working-class midwives was muted.

Midwifery achievements, education and exclusion

Loudon notes the 'reverse social class connection' with maternal mortality in the 1920s and 1930s: 'Social class was a much weaker determinant of mortality than the type of birth attendant' (1997: 185). He describes the achievements of midwives particularly in 'the delivery of the poor in their own homes'. From statistical analysis he concludes 'it was not so much the place of delivery as the type of birth attendant which was crucial; for it seems that trained midwives were more effective as attendants at normal labour than doctors...in Britain between 1850 and 1950 the midwife was the safer birth attendant for normal deliveries' (ibid.: 186–7).

In the interests of public health, the private practice of midwifery was increasingly marginalised by subsidised maternity care. The 1936 Midwives Act created a municipally salaried midwifery service and, very late in the day, the Institute came to support the efforts which led to this Act. The resulting district midwives lived, worked and became important figures in their district. Although, as single professional women, they were socially separated from their clients, they endeavoured in many ways to help them (Allison 1996).

The 1936 Midwives Act facilitated the extension of the midwife's work into antenatal care as well as creating a salaried service. This situation made it possible for the Central Midwives' Board to extend midwifery training, which it was hoped would attract a 'higher type into midwifery' (*Nursing Notes*, April 1932).

The efforts to raise the tone of midwifery by raising the training required of entrants continued through the rest of the twentieth century and is now demonstrated in the arguments for a graduate profession. As with the bona fide midwives, there is no evidence that clinical care provided by midwives without certificates, diplomas or degrees has different outcomes from that provided by their more educated colleagues. Yet the professional imperative continues: a need to raise the tone of midwifery and keep up with other professions. To say this is not to oppose education for midwives but to highlight the way in which raising educational standards was often used to scapegoat those with lesser/earlier qualifications. Indeed, this can be seen today in disputes as to whether highly experienced, non-graduate, clinical midwives can act as clinical mentors for undergraduate student midwives.

Institutionalisation and its effects

Loudon (1996, 1997) demonstrates that institutionalised birth could be a 'a massive obstetric disaster in terms of maternal mortality' (Marland and Rafferty 1997). Though evidence of this was available earlier this century, 'this evidence was apparently disbelieved or its significance rejected as repugnant to theoretical reasoning when further developments of the maternity services were organised' (Tew 1986). The fruits of such theoretical reasoning and the power of the medical profession are reflected in the official recommendations and statistics for place of birth.

During the second half of the twentieth century, normal birth, previously regarded as the midwife's field, moved into the hospital. There all pregnancies fell under medical management and came to be seen as 'normal only in retrospect'. This phrase, originally used by obstetricians (Percival 1970), was soon to be used by the Central Midwives Board in describing *The Role of the Midwife* (Central Midwives Board 1983). A 'scientific redefinition' of birth (De Vries 1996) had occurred, 'medical science' had become the 'predominant source of the social constructs of the culture of childbirth' (Oakley 1993) as the Church had been in the Middle Ages.

The institutionalisation of childbearing also demonstrates the shift in cultural codes of gender (Davies 1995) in maternity care. Traditionally the work of women, 'with women' in the privacy of the home, midwifery fitted well the culturally coded female skills in 'the maintenance of relationships and the sustenance of human life' (Bologh 1990). Organisational life, on the other hand, developed from social constructions of masculinity, coded as separating, controlling, competitive, masterful and hierarchy-orientated (Davies 1995). This analysis can be applied to the early twentieth-century tensions between caring for clients as individuals and the pressures towards professionalisation (Kirkham 1996a). Later, tensions were felt between the supportive care of individual childbearing women and the organisation of the institutions within which they bore their children.

Hospitals embody a 'hierarchy of institutional expertise' (Freidson 1970) which structures the experience of 'patients' and the subordinate professions for whom the dominant profession has the power to define. Midwives are low in the hierarchy, and their position is often seen as that of 'subcontractor' (Schwartz 1990) to 'medicine as the engineer repairing faulty machinery' (Littlewood and McHugh 1997), with all the 'separation of individuals from their wider social environment' (Doyal 1995) implied by that model of medicine. The female gendered skills of support, caring and being with women tend to be invisible within such gendered institutions. This is ironic, as so many working-class women in the 1940s and 1950s sought a hospital birth for a brief respite of rest and care in a life of unremitting toil.

Language, knowledge and technology

Language structures our experience, gives meaning to our perceptions and, at the same time, limits our thinking to ideas and concepts which our language can express. 'Language is a guide to social reality' (Sapir 1928). It is therefore not surprising that language is gendered and 'English is biased in favour of the male in both syntax and semantics' (Spender 1980), as well as being used very differently by men and women (Tannen 1991, 1995). The technical language in maternity care – and the one in which midwifery is taught – is that of obstetrics. Obstetric terminology is concerned with physical measurement and has no terms to describe the experience of childbearing women or the support and communication skills of midwifery. Such a linguistic situation ensures that official documents, or even the student curriculum, may take for granted, but do not conceptualise and therefore cannot acknowledge or transmit, basic midwifery skills. Thus, around birth, midwives and mothers become a 'muted group' (Hardman 1973):

> whose members become muted or are relatively less articulate compared with the dominant group because they have to express themselves through the structures and idioms of that group. It is not that muted groups can't speak but that they can't be heard.
>
> (Astbury 1996: 26)

As language structures experience, it provides a medium through which midwives have internalised the values of medicine and long since ceased to experience their situation as one of exclusion. Midwives acquire the language of their training and workplace and do not experience it as foreign to their needs. On non-obstetric issues their voice is muted. This situation is ironic as medical research now demonstrates the positive, measurable outcomes of the continuing presence of a 'supportive female companion' with labouring women (MIDIRS 1996). Knowledge of the means by which these outcomes are achieved awaits further research.

The pressure towards professionalisation has also produced a need to develop a body of knowledge to which access is limited and controlled by the profession. Midwifery knowledge developed rapidly, largely because of the growing technical complexity of obstetrics, whose front-line worker was the midwife. Knowledge of physiology and of medicine is important for safe practice. There is also a body of knowledge and skill that has been delegated by medicine: 'innovations by doctors which once routinised are then delegated to nurses or other paramedical occupations' (Hughes 1971). In Jennifer Sleep's view:

these newly acquired skills do not represent midwifery innovations prompted and directed by the needs of normally labouring
women. Many are developed as a consequence of practitioners'
frustration and consumer dissatisfaction and as such provide a
means of reducing the time spent waiting for junior doctors to
make and implement clinical decisions.

(Sleep 1992: 1467)

Dingwall *et al.* (1988) cautioned:

this downward delegation of routinised, albeit skilled, medical
tasks is at the expense of the [midwives'] role as a spiritual, or in
modern times, psychological support for the mother.

Not only is there less time, and less status, for the traditional support
skills, but the values of the delegating profession are implicit in the
delegated tasks.

The growth of obstetric technology profoundly affected power
relationships in other ways:

There is a hidden function of the tools of the trade...to do with
their symbolic function as indicators and enforcers of the social
distribution of knowledge and power to act in childbirth....
High technology, thus, draws in its wake a hierarchical distribution of knowledge and social authority that reflects the equally
hierarchical social position of birth attendants in medicalised
settings.

(Jordan 1987: 37)

Thus the woman is on the professionals' territory surrounded by
equipment that only they can interpret. The midwife often appears to
take the role of machine operative, and the woman that of the
container within which technology investigates the foetus. In the use
of technology there are also rituals which give staff a sense of control
even when the ritual is maintained in the face of contrary research
evidence, as is often the case with continuous electronic foetal heart
monitoring (Chalmers *et al.* 1989, Southern 1997). Such rituals,
whilst they may give staff a comforting, if false, sense of control,
deny any control to the childbearing woman. Thus the woman, who
is not ill, is excluded from playing a part in, as well as taking any
control over, her care.

Monitoring symbolises a fundamental change in the obstetric view of childbearing. It concerns all pregnancies and, compared with a statistical assessment of risk, normality seems a crude and possibly irrelevant concept.

Monitoring and surveillance deal with the problem of residual normalcy by ignoring it. Under this new regime no distinctions between normal and abnormal exist.

(Arney 1982: 85)

Obstetrics has moved from a defined area of abnormal childbearing to a much wider view, whilst at the same time accommodating demands from consumers for alternatives to the traditional medical model of birth:

The social organisation of obstetrics extended outwards from the hospital over large areas, putting in place a flexible system of obstetrical alternatives as it went. Even so, every aspect of birth became more carefully controlled, a structure of control I call 'monitoring' was deployed across a greatly expanded obstetrical space.

(ibid.: 9)

There is no midwifery equivalent of the 'flexible system of obstetrical alternatives'. By Arney's analysis, obstetrics has, in outgrowing its role of concern with the abnormal, threatened the adjacent role of concern with the normal. It could, therefore, be argued that, with the erosion of the limited role assigned to her in 1902, as the midwife's technical skill increased, her limited professional autonomy waned. As pregnancies are monitored for deviations from a normality which technical advances continuously redefine, new sets of values are internalised by midwives, who play a key role in making the resulting changes in care acceptable to mothers.

Expert knowledge and status have fundamentally changed midwives' relationships with childbearing women. Traditionally knowledge was shared between midwives and mothers. Jordan (1983) described traditional Maya midwives facilitating decision-making through the sharing of relevant stories by all the women present at a labour. All the knowledge there was made accessible and available to the labouring woman and her supporters, a very different situation from that of professional knowledge encoded in technical language with very different power relationships around decision-making.

An oppressed group

Midwifery in Britain, defined to such an extent by the more powerful profession of medicine, fits the definition of an oppressed group (Roberts 1983) as one 'which is controlled by societal forces that have determined its leadership behaviour'. The analysis of Freire (1972) gives insight into how, in the process of internalising the values of the more powerful group, the original characteristics of an oppressed group come to be negatively valued. This was clearly demonstrated as technical knowledge increased in the midwifery curriculum at the expense of traditional skills of support and empowerment, which had been conveyed to students as the 'situated knowledge' (Lave and Wenger 1991) of skilled midwives practising relatively autonomously. Midwifery insights were therefore muted or denied, with damaging effects for those who thereby rejected value in their own traditions and identity. The resulting low self-esteem is highly self-destructive (Taylor 1996), especially as it is held in balance with subservience to the more powerful group (Kirkham 1996b). The tension thus produced was seen by Fanon (1963) as released in 'horizontal violence': conflict within the oppressed group especially towards those seen as slightly deviant, which in turn reinforces the status quo. Such 'horizontal violence' has been described in very diverse midwifery settings (Brodie 1996a and 1996b, Leap 1997, Stapleton *et al.* 1998).

Oppressed groups also experience fear of change. This is often manifest around changes in midwifery and, sadly, has been frequently demonstrated around attempts in recent years to give choice and control to women with regard to their maternity care. Whilst some midwives have been keen to implement innovations, many pilot projects have been surrounded by resistance to change (see, for example, McCourt and Page 1996, Henderson 1997).

Thus midwives were not simply excluded from some areas of practice, though that undoubtedly happened. Educated and working as an oppressed group and internalising the values of medicine, they were excluded from professional confidence, autonomy and the ability to challenge. They became dependent upon obstetrics (Robinson 1990).

During the 1990s, however, midwives have put considerable effort into renegotiating their relationship with medicine, and there has been considerable goodwill in some areas of obstetrics for such renegotiation. Nevertheless, the reactions of an oppressed group are difficult to cast off. This is compounded by the extent to which midwives in some NHS settings now feel themselves to be oppressed by general management (Stapleton *et al.* 1998).

The culture of midwifery

The culture of midwifery within the NHS is one of a female oppressed group. Midwives continue in their efforts to support and care for childbearing women. Yet, as these efforts are not priorities of the institutions within which midwives work, they are not officially valued or rewarded. Neither are efforts made to sustain the skills of the caring aspect of the midwife's role. A dedication to selfless caring, therefore, continues alongside efforts to fulfil the expectations of the more powerful professions of medicine and latterly management, as well as meeting the needs of clients and raising the professional status of midwifery. Thus the midwife seeks to please in an increasing number of different directions with little to sustain her in these efforts. In such situations defence mechanisms are inevitable and can be manifest in resistance to change, horizontal violence, scapegoating and bullying (RCM 1996, Leap 1997, Stapleton *et al.* 1998).

The midwife and the childbearing woman

As women carry out most of the many acts which constitute maternity care, so they act out its changes. As the move from midwife to male practitioner resulted from a change in the culture of women, so a change in the employment of women staffed the maternity wards and created the maternity patient. Whilst most childbearing until the mid-1950s remained in the home, the woman retained the control associated with her own surrounding even if the midwife enforced firm ideas about the conduct of labour (Leap and Hunter 1993). With hospitalisation, the woman was on the territory of the professionals and her situation was much more closely controlled throughout her hospital stay.

The control of information

Ignorance of the process of labour and delivery made childbirth frightening whatever the setting for labour (Llewelyn Davies 1977). In hospital women also needed knowledge of how birth was managed, how staff behaved and what staff expected of them within the institution. In antenatal care and antenatal classes the midwife prepared women for hospitalisation as well as for childbirth.

Admission in labour was a process of institutionalisation and 'teaching the patient to be patient' (Kirkham 1983a). Women in labour are admitted to single rooms in which they gain relative privacy but lack the information about their setting which most new hospital patients learn from other patients. They are thus highly dependent upon staff, whose cues they heed closely, and who teach them, by word and action, the behaviour expected of a good patient (Kirkham 1983a and 1983b).

Whilst women are very dependent upon staff, as the only source of the information they need to orientate themselves to their labour, information is not given according to need. The giving of information is closely linked to the social class of the labouring woman. Whilst all women seek information (Green *et al.* 1988), women of higher social class are given more information (Cartwright 1979, Shapiro *et al.* 1983), as they are likely to be perceived as trustworthy in terms of their use of that information and to pose no threat to the equilibrium of staff (Kirkham 1983b). Despite midwives' desire to give information and their awareness of women's information needs, midwives feel the need to maintain the 'sentimental order of the ward' (Glaser and Strauss 1968). The maintenance of this order enhances the staff's control over their work and makes them feel more secure (Kirkham 1983b). Whilst the exercise of such control by staff may be understandable in terms of the pressures upon them, 'information represents power in the struggle for control and is thus a pivotal question in the study of negotiated order' (Rosenthal *et al.* 1980). In maternity care, power tends to stay with those who are used to exercising it. Midwives, excluded from exercising power in so many areas, tend to retain what little control they have, which is over the behaviour of clients, whose experience they are often seen as policing (Kirkham 1983b, Dearling 1997).

The inverse care law in midwifery

Perinatal mortality and morbidity is social class related (ONS 1996), and the difference between social classes has widened in recent years (Tyler 1994). There is evidence to suggest that the quality of maternity care is also social class linked in 'that the availability of good care tends to vary inversely with the need of the population served' (Tudor Hart 1971). In 1979 Cartwright identified that 'women from social class V were less likely to experience intensive antenatal care'. A study of the antenatal care of 896 women in three London teaching hospitals concluded that 'the quality of care given to pregnant women is associated with social class' (Arnold 1987). In their study of 1,193 Australian women's antenatal care, Brown and Lumley concluded that

> While the majority of women were happy with their antenatal care, an inverse care law still applied: women whose economic and social circumstances meant that they were most likely to need 'care' from caregivers were more likely to be limited in their choice of caregivers and to be dissatisfied with the care they received.
>
> (1993: 95)

It is perhaps not surprising that the majority of these women were happy with their care, as expectations are built from what is seen as possible. Women from deprived backgrounds do not maintain a burning awareness of exclusion but judge their present experience by what the past has led them to believe is possible. In antenatal classes, Cliff and Deery (1997) found 'a clear hierarchy in attendance...based on social class'. A study of women's experience of labour in a midwife-led unit found '[t]hose with the greatest need for support and continuity of care and carer are among those least likely to receive it' (Walker *et al.* 1995).

Poor obstetric outcomes are linked with ethnic group as well as social class (ONS 1996). Yet, rather than providing excellent care to these vulnerable women, maternity care for women from ethnic minorities tends to be insensitive, based upon stereotypes and unresponsive to the needs of individuals (Bowler 1993, Baxter 1996). The knowledge upon which midwives base this care is also likely to be inadequate (Dyson *et al.* 1996, Neille 1997). There is also evidence which suggests that maternity care is changing away from meeting the needs of some ethnic minority women (Bowes and Domokos 1996). Their social position as well as their experience of racism ensures that these women's expectations are low and their voices are unlikely to be heard. Childbearing women from many different minority groups are likely to receive maternity care which is inappropriate to their particular needs (Kargar and Hunt 1997).

The inverse care law is a phenomenon seen throughout medical care, and it is not surprising that it is seen clearly in maternity care, where medicine has expanded so greatly and midwives have internalised the values of medicine. Nevertheless, it is significant that this is an area where the vast majority of those involved are not ill and which produces a situation where those likely to have problems are relatively neglected despite the fact that the justification for the expansion of medical services was to detect deviations from the normal.

Recent changes and continuing patterns

In recent years there have been pressures for a fundamental change in the values underpinning maternity care and in its organisation. These pressures have come largely from childbearing women using a growing body of research evidence to support their aims. The result has been a range of radical changes towards partnership between childbearing women and midwives in a number of countries (Donley 1997). There are impressive publications on the partnership of midwives and mothers in countries such as New Zealand (see, for example, Guilliland and Pairman 1995).

The Winterton Report (HMSO 1992) and *Changing Childbirth* (DOH 1993) stress choice and control for women in their care and continuity of care so that they can form relationships with a small number of midwives and work in partnership with them. There is, therefore, a real sense in which midwives, seeking to meet the aims of *Changing Childbirth*, are trying to forge relationships with clients which are very different from those of the NHS and much nearer to the relationships which their pre-professional predecessors took for granted. The pressures that moved midwifery away from such relationships, however, still remain, and in some respects these pressures have been compounded.

Within the NHS, there have been numerous pilot schemes to evaluate ways in which the principle of partnership can be put into practice, often with impressive outcomes (e.g. McCourt and Page 1996). Nevertheless, pressure upon the funding of such projects, limited support from management (Bradshaw and Bradshaw 1997) and from obstetricians and GPs (Henderson 1997) has led to the end of many of these projects. This has led, in some places to a lowering of the impetus to improve care and a fear of change, partly because of the resistance which it can produce (Page 1997).

There is also a growing awareness that the implementation of *Changing Childbirth* (DOH 1993) can just fit in with the inverse care law (Tudor Hart 1971):

> In midwifery terms, there is a paradox of plenty which could, if unchecked, be made worse by the *Changing Childbirth* recommendations...It would be very sad indeed if *Changing Childbirth*

led only to healthy, well-educated and well-motivated women who consume more of the midwifery resources at the expense of those who arguably need them most. Midwives must recognise that choice is limited by circumstances and that the psychosocial effects of poverty mean that it is the most vulnerable women who demand the least.

(Tyler 1994: 553)

There are fundamental problems in implementing projects which are built upon different basic values from those of the surrounding medical system. An evaluation of women's experiences of maternity services in East London found that:

The observation that women want more information in order to make informed choice has been made for some time...Women with partners of lower social class are less likely to get the information that they want...There were...important socio-economic determinants of continuity [of carer]. Those women whose first language was English were nearly twice as likely to experience continuity as those with other first languages.

(Hemingway *et al.* 1994: 40, 42)

The inverse care law thus appears to be pernicious. There are problems for midwives too in seeking such radical change:

When New Zealand domiciliary midwives were seen to be taking the side of women in support of the midwifery model, we were criticised as being unprofessional. We were publicly accused of lowering the standards of the profession. At a midwives' seminar one midwife argued that a midwife's first loyalty was to her profession, while I maintained that it was to the women we attended. Those different concepts of loyalty are really about power relations.

(Donley 1997: 45)

It is, however, significant that these problems are now being debated locally and internationally. An International Confederation of Midwives meeting in 1996,

recognised as a major issue the need to strengthen partnership of women and midwives. It also acknowledged the need to raise the political consciousness of midwives. The latter need was obvious because internationally the majority of midwives was not quite ready to let go of its professional status and power which is dependent on a captive clientele within a bureaucracy.

(ibid.: 46)

Whilst such change is fraught with problems, there is clear evidence of progress and issues are being debated now which would not have been publicly discussed a few years ago. Evaluations of projects working in partnership with women have shown a change in the primary loyalty of the midwives towards those women rather than their employer or profession (Brodie 1996a). This can, in turn, create problems, including resistance to change and horizontal violence amongst midwives working adjacent to such projects (Brodie 1996b, Henderson 1997). Such response can create a 'fear of excellence' (Page 1997).

Another area of change which supports innovations in midwifery is that of research and the moves towards evidence-based practice. Research is now being used to challenge some areas of technological ritual in obstetrics. It is encouraging to read an article in a midwifery journal which starts: 'The best weapons childbirth practitioners have in the battle to improve maternity care is that the data are all on our side' (Goer 1997: 27).

Publications such as *Effective Care in Pregnancy and Childbirth* (Chalmers *et al.* 1989) and the *Cochrane Database of Systematic Reviews* (1995) make such 'weapons' available to midwives. Publications such as *Obstetric Myths Versus Research Realities* (Goer 1995) and efforts to help childbearing women gain the skills to appraise research reports critically (CASP 1997) all serve to aid midwives and women to work together in partnership.

Reviewing the evaluations of recent innovative midwifery projects, Lesley Page highlights the advantages of providing continuity of carer and concludes, 'The message which is coming through from the research is that what is best for mothers may also be best for midwives' (1997: 652)

Though change is still at a very early stage, there are signs of change in language and in the naming of states of exclusion for midwives and childbearing women. The concept of muting is an important example of a term used for the lack of voice of mothers with consequent damaging effects (Brown *et al.* 1994, Bowes and Domokos 1996, Littlewood and McHugh 1997) which went on to be used in describing the similar position of midwives (Stapleton *et al.* 1998). The naming of such concepts makes communication and subsequent action possible.

Research can be seen as 'anti-authoritarian' in its nature (Chalmers 1983) and as:

> fostering a greater sense of uncertainty in our approach to care: admitting that 'we do not know' can provide an impetus to the discovery and evaluation of ways in which practice can be improved.
>
> (Sleep 1992: 1468)

Such uncertainty is, however, highly uncomfortable and threatening to midwives who have adjusted over whole careers to NHS midwifery practice, which is controlled and therefore relatively certain, if limiting and oppressive. It must also be borne in mind that the economic imperative, which drives much of the present demand for research evidence, has very different origins from that of the partnership between midwives and mothers. The model of health care which sees service users as consumers has also been a factor in producing some of the encouraging trends in current maternity care. Nevertheless, consumerisation has also left midwives with a fear of litigation which can produce defensive practice. Hospital management has also, in some places, responded to consumerism in ways which leave midwives fearful and threatened, limited in their practice and spending a large amount of time filling in critical incident forms (Stapleton *et al.* 1998). Whilst it has made initial change possible, there must be a limit to how far the concept of a consumer can continue to be useful with regard to life's most productive act.

Nevertheless, childbearing women in New Zealand and some parts of Canada have galvanised midwives into action in partnership with them which led to changed legislation and changed practice. There are signs that similar change is possible in this country. Efforts are being made, by both lay groups and midwives, to make sensitive and responsive midwifery care possible for groups of women who have previously been excluded. It is now possible that, rather than midwives being expert, professional and oppressed, the future of British midwifery could be, once again, with women.

References

Allison, J. (1996) *Delivered at Home*, London: Chapman and Hall.

Arney, W.R. (1982) *Power and the Profession of Obstetrics*, Chicago: University of Chicago Press.

Arnold, M. (1987) 'The cycle of maternal deprivation', *Midwife, Health Visitor and Community Nurse* 23, 12: 539–42.

Astbury, J. (1996) *Crazy for You: The Making of Women's Madness*, Melbourne: Oxford University Press.

Baxter, C. (1996) 'Working from a multiracial perspective', in D. Kroll (ed.) *Midwifery Care for the Future*, London: Baillière Tindall.

Blumenfeld-Kosinski, R. (1990) *Not of Woman Born: Representations of Caesarean Birth in Medieval and Renaissance Culture*, Ithaca: Cornell University Press.

Bologh, R.W. (1990) *Love or Greatness: Max Weber and Masculine Thinking – a Feminist Inquiry*, London: Unwin Hyman.

Bowes, A.M. and Domokos, T.M. (1996) 'Pakistani women and maternity care: raising muted voices', *Sociology of Health and Illness* 18, 1: 45–65.

Bowler, I. (1993) 'They're not the same as us: midwives' stereotypes of South Asian descent maternity patients', *Sociology of Health and Illness* 15, 2: 157–78.

Bradshaw, M.G. and Bradshaw, P.L. (1997) 'Changing childbirth – the midwifery managers' tale', *Journal of Nurse Management* 5, 143–9.

Brodie, P. (1996a) 'Australian team midwives in transition', paper presented to International Confederation of Midwives, 24th Triennial Conference, Oslo.

——(1996b) 'Being with women: the experience of Australian team midwives', unpublished Masters thesis, University of Technology, Sydney, Australia.

Brown, S. and Lumley, J. (1993) 'Antenatal care: a case of the inverse care law?', *Australian Journal of Public Health* 17, 2: 95–103.

Brown, S., Lumley, J., Small, R. and Astbury, J. (1994) *Missing Voices: The Experience of Motherhood*, Melbourne: Oxford University Press.

Campbell, J.M. (1924) *Maternal Mortality Associated with Childbearing*, London: HMSO.

Cartwright, A. (1979) *The Dignity of Labour*, London: Tavistock.

CASP (1997) *CASP for MSLCs: A Project Enabling Maternity Service Liaison Committees to Develop an Evidence Based Approach to Changing Childbirth*, London: CASP.

Central Midwives Board (1983) *The Role of the Midwife*, Norwich: Hymns Ancient and Modern.

Chalmers, I. (1983) 'Scientific enquiry and authoritarianism in prenatal care and education', *Birth* 10, 151–6.

Chalmers, I., Enkin, M. and Keirse, M.J.N.C. (eds) (1989) *Effective Care in Pregnancy and Childbirth*, Oxford: Oxford University Press.

Cliff, D. and Deery, R. (1997) 'Too much like school: social class, age, marital status and attendance/non-attendance at antenatal classes', *Midwifery* 13, 139–45.

Cochrane Database of Systematic Reviews (1995), London: BMJ Publishing.

Cox, C. (1982) 'Where are we now?', *Midwives Chronicle*, January: 3–6.

Davies, C. (1995) *Gender and the Professional Predicament In Nursing*, Buckingham: Open University Press.

Davis, C. (1983) 'Professional strategies as time- and culture-bound: American and British nursing circa 1893', in E.C. Langeman (ed.) *Nursing History: New Perspectives, New Possibilities*, New York: Teachers College Press.

Dearling, J. (1997) 'Is it a fair cop? Midwives as health police in breast-feeding promotion', *Midwives* 110, 1319: 296.

Department of Health (DOH) (1993) *Changing Childbirth*, London: HMSO.

De Vries, R.G. (1996) *Making Midwives Legal*, Columbus: Ohio State University Press.

Dingwall, R., Rafferty, A.M. and Webster, C. (1988) *An Introduction to the Social History of Nursing*, London: Routledge, Chapman and Hall.

Donley, J. (1997) 'Reclaiming partnership in birth', *Midwifery Today* 43, 45–69.

Donnison, J. (1977) *Midwives and Medical Men: A History of Inter-professional Rivalries and Women's Rights*, London: Heinemann.

Doyal, L. (1995) *What Makes Women Sick?*, London: Macmillan.

Dyson, S.M., Fielder, A.V. and Kirkham, M.J. (1996) 'Midwives' and senior student midwives' knowledge of haemoglobinopathies in England', *Midwifery* 12, 23–30.

Elliot, P. (1972) *The Sociology of Professions*, New York: Macmillan.

Etzioni, A. (ed.) (1969) *The Semi-Professions and their Organisation*, New York: Free Press.

Fanon, F. (1963) *The Wretched of the Earth*, New York: Grove Press.

Freidson, E. (1970) *Professional Dominance: The Social Structure of Medical Care*, Chicago: Aldine.

Freire, P. (1972) *The Pedagogy of the Oppressed*, Harmondsworth: Penguin.

Glaser, B.G. and Strauss, A.L. (1968) *Time for Dying*, Chicago: Aldine.

Goer, H. (1995) *Obstetric Myths Versus Research Realities: A Guide to the Medical Literature*, Westport, Connecticut: Bergin and Garvey.

——(1997) 'How to use the medical literature for fun and profit', *Midwifery Today* 43, 27.

Green, J.M., Coupland, V. and Kitzinger, J.V. (1988) *Great Expectations: A Prospective Study of Women's Expectations and Experiences of Child-birth*, Cambridge: Child Care and Development Group, University of Cambridge.

Guilliland, K. and Pairman, S. (1995) *The Midwifery Partnership: A Model for Practice*, Wellington, New Zealand: Dept. of Nursing and Midwifery, Victoria University of Wellington.

Hardman, C. (1973) 'Can there be an anthropology of children?', *Journal of the Anthropological Society of Oxford* 4, 85–99.

Heagerty, B.V. (1990) 'Gender and professionalization: the struggle for British midwifery, 1900–1936', unpublished PhD thesis, Michigan State University (copy in Royal College of Midwives Library, London).

Hemingway, H., Saunders, D. and Parson, L. (1994) *Women's Experiences* of *Maternity Care in East London: An Evaluation*, London: Directorate of Public Health, ELCHA.

Henderson, C. (1997) '*Changing Childbirth' and the West Midlands Region*, London: Royal College of Midwives.

HMSO (1892) *Report from the Select Committee on the Registration of Midwives, House of Commons*, London: HMSO.

——(1992) *Parliamentary Select Committee on Health: Second Report on the Maternity Services*, London: HMSO.

Hughes, E.C. (1971) *The Sociological Eye*, Chicago: Aldine.

Isherwood, K.M. (1992) 'Are British midwives "with women"? – the evidence', *Midwifery Matters* 54, Autumn: 14–17.

Jordan, B. (1983) *Birth in Four Cultures*, Montreal: Eden Press.

——(1987) 'The hut and the hospital: information, power and symbolism in the artefacts of birth', *Birth* 14, 1: 36–40.

Kargar, I. and Hunt, S.C. (eds) (1997) *Challenges in Midwifery Care*, London: Macmillan.

Kirkham, M.J. (1983a) 'Admission in labour: teaching the patient to be patient?', *Midwives Chronicle* February: 44–5.

——(1983b) 'Labouring in the dark: limitations on the giving of information to enable patients to orientate themselves to the likely events and time-scale of labour', in J. Wilson-Barnett (ed.) *Nursing Research: Ten Studies in Patient Care*, Chichester: Wiley.

——(1989) 'Midwives and information-giving during labour', in S. Robinson and A.M. Thompson (eds) *Midwives, Research and Childbirth*, Vol. I, London: Chapman Hall.

——(1996a) 'Professionalisation past and present: with women or with the powers that be?', in D. Kroll (ed.) *Midwifery Care for the Future*, London: Baillière Tindall.

——(1996b) *Supervision of Midwives*, Hale: Books for Midwives.

Lave, J. and Wenger, E. (1991) *Situated Learning: Legitimate Peripheral Participation*, Cambridge: Cambridge University Press.

Leap, N. (1997) 'Making sense of horizontal violence in midwifery', *British Journal of Midwifery* 5, 11: 689.

Leap, N. and Hunter, B. (1993) *The Midwife's Tale*, London: Scarlett Press.

Littlewood, J. and McHugh, N. (1997) *Maternal Distress and Postnatal Depression*, London: Macmillan.

Llewelyn Davies, M. (ed.) (1977) *Life as We Have Known It: By Co-operative Working Women*, London: Virago.

Loudon, I. (1996) *Childbed Fever: A Documentary History*, New York: Garland Press.

——(1997) 'Midwives and the quality of maternal care', in H. Marland and A.M. Rafferty (eds) *Midwives, Society and Childbirth*, London: Routledge.

Marland, H. and Rafferty A.M. (eds) (1997) *Midwives, Society and Childbirth*, London: Routledge.

McCourt, C. and Page, L. (1996) *Report on the Evaluation of One-to-One*

Midwifery, London: Hammersmith Hospital and Thames Valley University.

MIDIRS and the NHS Centre for Reviews and Dissemination (1996) *Informed Choice for Professional: Support in Labour*, Bristol: MIDIRS.

Neille, E. (1997) 'Control for Black and ethnic minority women: a meaningless pursuit', in M.J. Kirkham and E.R. Perkins (eds) *Reflections on Midwifery*, London: Baillière Tindall.

Nursing Notes was the journal of the Midwives Institute which later became the Royal College of Midwives. All issues of this journal can be found in the RCM library.

Oakley, A. (1993) *Essays on Women, Medicine and Health*, Edinburgh: Edinburgh University Press.

Office for National Statistics (ONS) (1996) *Population and Health Monitor*, DH3 96/3, London: ONS.

Page, L. (1997) 'Misplaced values: in fear of excellence', *British Journal of Midwifery* 5, 11: 652–4.

Percival, P. (1970) 'Management of normal labour', *The Practitioner* 1221: 204.

Radcliffe, W. (1967) *Milestones in Midwifery*, Bristol: Wright.

Roberts, S.J. (1983) 'Oppressed group behaviour: implications for nursing', *Advances in Nursing Science*, July: 21–30.

Robinson, S. (1990) 'Maintaining the independence of midwifery', in J. Garcia, R. Kilpatrick and M. Richards (eds) *The Politics of Maternity Care*, Oxford: Clarendon.

Rosenthal, C.J., Marshall, V.W., MacPherson, A.S. and French, S.E. (1980) *Nurses, Patients and Families*, London: Croom Helm.

Royal College of Midwives (1996) *In Place of Fear: Recognising and Confronting the Problem of Bullying in Midwifery*, London: The Royal College of Midwives.

Sandall, J. (1995) 'Choice, continuity and control: changing midwifery towards a sociological perspective', *Midwifery* 11, 4: 201–9.

Sapir, E. (1928) *Culture, Language and Personality*, (1966 edn) D.G. Mandlebaum (ed.), Berkley, California: University of California Press.

Schwarz, E.W. (1990) 'The engineering of childbirth: a new obstetric programme as reflected in British obstetric textbooks, 1969–1980', in J. Garcia, R. Kilpatrick and M. Richards (eds) *The Politics of Maternity Care*, Oxford: Clarendon.

Shapiro, M.C., Najman, J.M., Chang, A., Keeping, J.D., Morrison, J. and Western J.S. (1983) 'Information control and the exercise of power in the obstetrical encounter', *Social Science and Medicine* 17, 3: 139–46.

Simpson, R.I. and Simpson, I.H. (1969) 'Women and bureaucracy in the semi-professions', in A. Etzioni (ed.) *The Semi-Professions and their Organisation*, New York: Free Press.

Sleep, J. (1992) 'Research and the practice of midwifery', *Journal of Advanced Nursing* 17, 1465–71.

Smith, F.B. (1979) *The People's Health 1830–1910*, London: Croom Helm.

Southern, J. (1997) 'Talking with Robbie Davis-Floyd', *Midwifery Today* 43: 13.

Spender, D. (1980) *Man-Made Language*, London: Routledge and Kegan Paul.

Stapleton, H., Duerden J. and Kirkham, M. (1998) *Evaluation of the Impact of the Supervision of Midwives on Professional Practice and the Quality of Midwifery Care*, London: ENB.

Tannen, D. (1991) *You Just Don't Understand: Women and Men in Conversation*, London: Virago.

——(1995) *Talking from 9 to 5: Women and Men at Work: Language, Sex and Power*, London: Virago.

Taylor, M. (1996) 'An ex-midwife's reflections on supervision', in M. Kirkham (ed.) *Supervision of Midwives*, Hale: Books for Midwives.

Tew, M. (1978) 'The case against hospital deliveries: the statistical evidence', in S. Kitzinger and J. Davis (eds) *The Place of Birth*, Oxford: Oxford University Press.

——(1986) 'The practice of birth attendants and the safety of birth', *Midwifery* 2, 1: 3–10.

Tudor Hart, J. (1971) 'The inverse care law', *The Lancet* 27 February: 405–12.

Tyler, S. (1994) 'Maternity care and the paradox of plenty', *British Journal of Midwifery* 2, 11: 552–4.

Walker, J.M., Hall, S. and Thomas, M. (1995) 'The experience of labour: a perspective from those receiving care in a midwife-led unit', *Midwifery* 11, 120–9.

Wilkinson, R.G. (1996) *Unhealthy Societies*, London: Routledge.

Willughby, P. (1972) *Observations in Midwifery*, Wakefield: SR Publishers.

Wilson, A. (1995) *The Making of Man-midwifery: Childbirth in England 1660–1771*, London: UCL Press.

Witz, A. (1992) *Professions and Patriarchy*, London: Routledge.

World Health Organisation (WHO) (1965) *The Midwife in Maternity Care: Report of a WHO Expert Committee*, Geneva: World Health Organisation.

6 Social exclusion and madness

The complicity of psychiatric medicine and nursing

Peter Alan Morrall

Introduction

> The history of madness is the history of power...It requires power to control it. Threatening the normal structures of authority, insanity is engaged in an endless dialogue...about power.
>
> (Porter 1987: 39)

Since ancient times the powerful, whether regarded as a unitary and privileged 'class' or as disconnected groupings dispersed throughout society, have attempted to maintain social order by exercising control over those deemed 'irrational'. Over two millennia, 'reason' has ascended as the overriding ideology, and has been used to justify the existence of stability in Western society. Rationality and reasonableness form the fundamental tenets of the industrial ('modernist') epoch. Mental disorder in the individual has come to be viewed as placing in jeopardy the 'health' of society as a whole. It is the claim of 'rationalism' that unhealthy societies will disintegrate and collapse eventually into civil war (Porter 1987).

Madness intimidates the powerful because unintelligible actions and oratory are flaunted in the public arena. The naked hysteric running through the city centre, the agitated ramblings of the neurotic in the workplace, or the paranoid schizophrenic killing an innocent bystander, are puissant reminders to authority of the danger posed by the mentally ill. The very credibility and perpetuity of the 'rationalist' paradigm is undermined by the 'crazed' behaviour and thinking of the insane.

In this chapter I examine how psychiatry and psychiatric nursing collaborate in the governance of the mentally disordered on behalf of the state. Specifically, I review the notion of power and rationality in society. I discuss also the apotheosis of social exclusion, the asylum.

Asylumdom, an ongoing period in which custodial warehouses have been used to 'store' sections of the population considered to be 'unreasonable' (Scull 1993), represents an ostentatious display of 'the power to expel' by the state and psychiatry.

Power

> For some theorists, power is inevitably concentrated and centralized in modern society, in a monolithic way, while others view it as widely distributed and continuously contested, in a pluralist way.
>
> (Waters 1994: 219)

The complex nature of power produces problems in attempting to identify where and in whom power is located (Porter 1996). Power in society can be conceptualised as being either structured or diffused and amorphous. That is, on the one hand, power is accumulated by certain sections of society (especially the state and its representative institutions). On the other hand, power pervades all areas of social life (including that of the professional practice of psychiatric medicine and mental health nursing), and alters its site and potency over time.

Moreover, power is linked inextricably to resources (Dowding 1996). The notion of 'resources' implies a multitude of interconnected factors, which influence each other on a number of different levels. For example, the power of an individual is affected by: her or his personal volition, knowledge, physical and intellectual capacities; the norms and mores of the institutions and social strata to which she or he belongs; and the degree to which particular organisations invest in her or him (for example, in the form of educational qualifications, pecuniary reward, or promotion). Social groups are also affected by resource factors, for example the property (either as residential or commercial estate) or prestige they acquire. In capitalist society, the relationship between ownership and social status is infallible.

For Dowding (1996) power can be conceived of as either the relatively simple and direct ability to bring about an intended outcome ('power to'), or the sophisticated skill to make something happen indirectly ('power over'). Power exists, therefore, when an individual behaves in such a way that will produce a change in another individual (Cartwright and Zander 1968). A psychiatric nurse has the legal power 'to' prevent a compulsorily detained patient (and under certain conditions, a voluntary patient) from leaving the hospital ward. A therapist using, for example, cognitive-behavioural, rational-emotive, or psychoanalytic techniques can have power 'over' a client, so that the latter's conduct and feelings are modified insidiously.

The power of the psychotherapist is to some degree 'open' in the sense that the implications of entering into therapy are usually discussed with the client. Indeed, 'change' is the *sine qua non* of most psychotherapeutic philosophies, and a declared acceptance of this principle is demanded from the client. However, psychotherapy is in essence deceitful, as the full significance of the therapist's potential to influence is invariably not comprehended by the client (Smail 1984). Paradoxically, an inability on the part of the therapist to transform the social, economic and political conditions, which (arguably) are the root cause of an individual's psychological problems (Masson 1992, Morrall 1998a), is seldom proclaimed.

Those with power, however, may not exhibit openly their powerful predilections at all:

> Power is a dispositional concept. To say that I have the power to throw a stone 50 metres is to say that I *could* throw that stone 50 metres, not that I *am* throwing it that far...Dispositional properties...refer to what might be and not necessarily to what is...The problem for studying power is that we may have to discover the power of actors without actually seeing them wield that power.
>
> (Dowding 1996: 3–4)

Furthermore, power is socially prescribed. That is, society confers high status and authority on individuals in particular roles: police officers, politicians, doctors, lawyers, judges. Power is gained also through the acquiescence of others. For example, for a medical practitioner to be dominant in the doctor–patient relationship, the latter must adopt the passive 'sick role'. But power can be lost. In a consumer-oriented and market-driven social system it can be argued that there has been a demise of deference to traditional expertise and authority. Moreover, the enormous social and political upheavals in Eastern Europe, Albania, Yugoslavia and Zaire are examples of once powerful social systems being dislocated and replaced.

Structured power

From the structuralist perspective, society is stratified. A vital constituent of the structure of society is power. For Marxist theorists, power is expropriated by the section of society which owns the resources of production. In capitalist societies, the *bourgeoisie* (that is, the dominant class) have gained ownership of industry and commerce. The powerful interests of this 'class' permeate all social and political organisations, and human relationships. That is, the capitalist ideology infiltrates all aspects of an individual's personal and social life.

Moreover, as Lukes (1974) has observed, not only does the social system dictate what is on the menu of life, but what we believe should be on that menu in the first place is also fabricated for us. The desires of the mass of the population (for example, to have washing machines, new cars, exotic holidays, and even 'good health'), far from being under the free will of the individual, are fashioned by the capitalist class. We accept as 'normal' the work ethic, paid labour, material possession, and the legitimacy of the social hierarchy – all of which are necessary for the survival of the capitalist system:

> To ensure a skilled and willing labour force, workers [sic] need to be trained to acquire skills but they also need to be willing to accept their subordinate position in society.
>
> (Layder 1994: 40)

In the main, structuralist theory regards the state (government and political organisations; legal, health, and educational institutions) as a conduit for the interests of the dominant class. However, as Nicos Poulantzas (1978) has pointed out, the connection between the state and those with economic power may at times appear antithetical. For example, a government may institute laws which ensure a basic wage for employees, against the wishes of employers. However, the social system itself is not being dismantled in these circumstances, as the essential values and practices of capitalism remain intact. Furthermore, although professionals such as psychiatrists may not be aligned unequivocally with the dominant class, they (and their nursing co-collaborators) either directly or indirectly shore up the capitalist system through their association with the functions of the state.

Dispersed power

The post-structuralist approach, however, posits that power is factionalised. No one group maintains power constantly, and power is not focused in one segment of society (whether the state, an elite, or class) indefinitely. Subjugation is legitimised and reinforced essentially through language and associated symbols of power ('discourse') as well as by the application of rules restricting alternative types of actions (Waters 1994). Various collections of people (for example, political parties; corporate business; academic disciplines; the professions), create their own discourse and regulatory procedures.

Foucault (1971, 1973) explored how medical knowledge has been constructed to form an apparently authoritative perspective (or 'gaze'). He argues that what purports to be knowledge is the result of specific historical and social processes, rather than being 'factual', 'true', or the successful product of medical invention. Extreme relativism can, therefore, be seen to be the corollary of post-structuralist theory. That is, each society (as well as every power-laden social grouping) in every epoch, has a unique claim to comprehend 'reality': 'Different societies and different historical periods have different conventions and therefore different realities' (Turner 1995: 11).

This line of reasoning would imply that seemingly categorical entities such as 'health' and 'disease' are mere constructions. Diabetes, obesity, anorexia nervosa, hyperactivity, heart disease, dementia and schizophrenia become arbitrary classifications whose existence and boundaries are context-tied. Furthermore, the way in which human subjects think and talk about their bodies is controlled by the concepts, theories and symbols that have been supplied by the medical and para-medical professions.

The medical discourse in turn is a reflection of what society has deemed to be of significance at that point in time. Asking patients about their exercise, smoking and drinking habits, and encouraging them to take more responsibility for their health is not simply an example of good medical and nursing practice. The health care agenda is pre-set as a result of social, economic and political contingencies which act beneath the surface of user–professional encounters. Western ideas of health care are, for example, a consequence of such historical events as the Enlightenment and industrialisation. Events such as these have gradually shaped our understanding of what is valued in society away from religion and community responsibility towards an acceptance of the singularity and sanctity of the human 'body' (Brooks 1993).

Asylum

The response of the powerful to those perceived to be *non compos mentis* has been one of segregation and marginalisation. Asylums, built beyond the scrutiny of the 'normal' population, were material manifestations of exclusionary, beneficent and Darwinian convictions of the Victorian age.

Until the beginning of the nineteenth century, the mentally ill were in the main still cared for by their families (Scull 1993). However, thousands of mentally disordered people were contained, from the seventeenth century onwards, within houses of correction, private madhouses and local parish workhouses. They were victims of the pan-European 'Great Confinement' (Foucault 1971), which resulted in those who challenged the moral values of the bourgeois class being isolated from the rest of the population. These 'deviant' groups included the poor, the work-shy, the homeless and criminals. In Foucault's terms, 'reason' was separated from 'unreason'. Although the mentally ill were now no longer subjected to torture and execution, characteristic 'treatment' of the Middle Ages, the 'care' they received in these institutions was frequently appalling (Gallagher 1995).

Following the 1845 Lunacy Act in Britain, local authorities were forced to provide for the mentally ill through a massive public building programme. Along with the Poor Law Amendment Act of 1834, the 1845 act heralded the beginning of 'Victorian Asylumdom' – the segregation of the mentally ill into a centralised and unitary form of residence away from the rest of the community and other deviant populations (Foucault 1971, Scull 1979). This first 'psychiatric revolution' (Scull 1981) presented the opportunity for the profession of medicine (and nursing) to emerge as legitimate 'surveyors' of madness. That is, the medical profession was not instrumental in the creation of the asylum movement, but capitalised on a 'market opportunity':

> the sequestration of lunatics was primarily an expression of civil policy, more an initiative from magistrates, philanthropists and families than an achievement – for good or ill – of the doctors. Indeed, the rise of psychological medicine was more the consequence than the cause of the rise of the insane asylum. Psychiatry could flourish once, but not before, large numbers of inmates were crowded into asylums.
>
> (Porter 1987: 17)

It was the role of the psychiatrist as administrator, rather than that as a skilled and effective practitioner, which provided the opportunity for a power base to be established in the asylum (Scull 1993, Rogers and Pilgrim 1996).

From the later eighteenth century, 'moral treatment', supported by lay philanthropists and religious groups such as the Quakers, competed with the stimulants, sedatives, emetics, purgatives, bloodletting, cold and hot baths, and mechanical restraints of 'organic' psychiatry. Moral management invoked a more benevolent approach, which held that unreason could be brought back to reason if handled more humanely:

> This movement aimed in effect to revive the dormant humanity of the mad, by treating them as endowed with a residuum at least of normal emotions, still capable of excitation and training...They needed to be treated essentially like children, who required a stiff dose of rigorous discipline, rectification and retraining in thinking and training.
>
> (Porter 1987: 19)

In the early nineteenth century, the medical profession gained legal control over the asylums. Employing its well-used technique of 'inclusion', rather than attacking popular 'alternative' techniques, doctors encompassed moral treatment within their assortment of procedures. The effect of 'medicalising' moral treatment was to leave psychiatrists 'in charge of the whole enterprise' (Johnstone 1989: 177). By the time the 1890 Lunacy Act was instituted, the monopolisation of the care of the mentally ill by the medical profession enabled doctors to redefine the traditional category of 'madness' to that of 'mental illness' (Baruch and Treacher 1978). The medicalisation of one form of deviancy (mental disturbance) had been achieved.

After 1845, the keeper changed into the 'attendant'. The attendants were responsible for the general upkeep of the new institutions for the insane, but were to become 'the medical superintendent's servants, with primary responsibility to carry out his orders' (Nolan 1993: 6). Women who became attendants were in the main referred to as 'nurses'. It wasn't until the end of the nineteenth century that men were also accorded this title.

Psychiatry, as a branch of medicine, has presided over the mental health industry in Britain since the nineteenth century 'coup' over its rivals (Baruch and Treacher 1978). However, it has been suggested that the demise of the asylums as the locale for psychiatric care has resulted in the 'fragmentation' of medical dominance (Samson 1995). But Bean and Mounser argue cogently that the structural position of psychiatry has actually become more entrenched in the twentieth century. For Bean and Mounser, psychiatry, far from being undermined, has spread into the community and augmented its retinue of allied disciplines:

> Psychiatrists have exchanged their traditional power-base in mental hospitals to expand into general hospitals alongside the physicians and the surgeons, as well as out into the community to encroach on the GPs' domain presenting themselves as 'experts' in the care of the mentally ill. They have expanded to present the world with an entourage – the multidisciplinary team, consisting of social workers, nurses, psychologists, behavioural therapists and occupational therapists. And these auxiliary staff now emulate the medical approach and in so doing reinforce the credibility of the *power* of psychiatry.
>
> (Bean and Mounser 1993: 168)

Although other occupational groups (especially clinical psychology) may engage in professional rivalry, and can claim some measure of success, psychiatry has not as yet relinquished substantially its influence on the praxis and ideology of mental health care.

Decarceration and recarceration

When the policy of incarcerating the mentally disordered *en masse* in the countryside became untenable, slum housing, prisons and the streets of the city provided alternative accommodation to be shared with other groups on the periphery of society. With 'care in the community' has come an exponential upsurge in the ghettoisation and neglect of the mentally ill. Specifically, there has been a substantial rise in the number of mentally ill people who live in squalor, are homeless, reside in bed-and-breakfast accommodation, are jailed, and who have joined the ranks of the long-term unemployed (Murphy 1991, Audit Commission 1994, Craig *et al.* 1995, Mihill 1995, Johnson *et al.* 1997; Bennetto 1998). For the mentally disturbed, the price for social integration has been profound social indifference.

However, although on the edge of society, the mentally ill have attracted too much public attention. The suicidal, violent and homicidal tendencies of a minority of the most seriously mentally distressed have increased the visibility of 'unreason'. Reaction has been widespread. A plethora of reports from pressure groups, inquiries, and the media have expressed rage about inadequate provision and, with some justification (Morrall 1997b), the 'lack of rigour' by mental health professionals and managers of the health services in executing control over the mentally ill:

> A series of errors were made in the care of a mental patient who went on to kill his neighbour, an independent report concluded yesterday...The report says [that the] death could not have been predicted. But it adds that [the patient] had received a poor standard of care, and vital information was not passed from one agency to another.
>
> (unattributed editorial, *Guardian*, 1998)

The mentally ill have been at risk of 'recarceration' throughout the era of 'care in the community' (Morrall 1987). That is, the opposition to de-institutionalisation has endured, with demands persisting for the Victorian asylums to be used again for the care of the mentally ill. Moreover, recognising the need for mentally disturbed people to have a place of refuge, some have called for asylumdom to be reintroduced, but this time within, rather than outside, the general population (Carrier and Tomlinson 1996). The 'New Labour' government of the United Kingdom, elected in 1997, appears to be reverting to a programme of incarceration, and preparing to establish more in-patient accommodation and build more 'secure units' for the mentally ill:

> The policy of sending mentally ill people out of hospital to be cared for in the community is to be reversed by the Government. Frank Dobson, the Health Secretary, said...that seriously disturbed psychiatric patients must be kept in secure units to protect the public.
>
> (Thompson and Sylvester 1998)

The re-establishment of institutional approaches is in tension with the focus on 'primary' care for health services proposed by a previous Conservative government (NHS Management Executive 1996, Timmins 1996) and approved by the subsequent Labour administration (DOH 1998a). Moreover, the announcement about secure units came merely a month after the British Prime Minister, Tony Blair, had launched a 'Social Exclusion Unit', designed to bring back into society elements of a growing underclass stranded in a cycle of deprivation, unable to engage in the mainstream social activities of being adequately employed, living in acceptable housing, and gaining appropriate education: 'New Labour was created so that we became the party of all the people; so that we could win power with the purpose of re-building Britain as one nation and giving everyone a stake in society' (Blair 1997).

It would appear that Blair's uncompromising language of social 'inclusion' has an implicit caveat in relation to the mentally disordered!

Social anarchy

The asylum, however, is an architectural and philosophical edifice of modernity. It exemplified the rationality of social engineering and scientific medicine. It was, after all, from the points of view of the Victorian eugenicist and bourgeois philanthropist, quite 'sensible' to protect society and the 'insensible' from each other. Psychiatry had a pre-packaged laboratory, with captive guinea pigs on whom therapeutic experimentation (whether 'moral', psychological, pharmaceutical or surgical) could be indulged with impunity.

Moreover, the birth of the asylum was as a consequence of the state implementing centralised social control measures (Scull 1993). It was not until the nineteenth century that the state could benefit from capitalist administrative *savoir-faire*, a necessary precondition for the consolidation of social control measures. Furthermore, capitalist enterprise demanded economic and social rationalism, signified (in part) by the exclusion of the socially disruptive. Consequently, there is an inviolable link between the expansion of capitalism, the state, and such exclusionary apparatus as the asylum.

In the modern age society has been viewed as being in a condition of perpetual progress. Rationalism (the belief in logical solutions to the problems of society), education, science and technology are considered to be producing a better world in which wars will have no purpose and therefore will not occur, affluence will be pandemic, and illness will be eradicated.

But the world since the late twentieth century has been going through a series of tumultuous transformations as established social structures react to techno-scientific revolutions, a reordering of previous economic arrangements between societies, the creation of globalised markets and communication systems, and a metamorphosis in cultural values:

> we may no longer be living under the aegis of an industrial capitalist culture which can tell us what is true, right and beautiful, and also what our place is in the grand scheme, but under a

chaotic, mass-mediated, individual-preference-based culture of postmodernism.

(Waters 1994: 206)

From this perspective, there are no a priori moral, fiscal, or political principles on which individual and social behaviour can be forged. In this revolutionary period, the institutions which nurtured human security in the past are dead, dying, or mutating. For example, there is no longer a perceived norm for the membership and organisation of society's core social grouping – the family. Political parties have ditched their historical ideological affiliations to particular sections of society in favour of 'pragmatic' solutions to each event or issue. Workers rarely have stable and long-term jobs, but face instead the prospect of vacillating career 'opportunities', and 'flexible' employment conditions. 'Authentic' health care now encompasses such disparate and epistemologically incompatible medical interventions as gene therapy, acupuncture, neural grafting, homoeopathy and psychoanalysis.

Moreover, there are no assurances that these new social arrangements will themselves be anything more than ephemeral. The practices of the family, politicians, workers and doctors may change in ways yet to be defined, or could revert to previous patterns. The postmodernist dictum, therefore, can be summed up as 'the only certainty is uncertainty'.

Incoherent services

The mental health industry itself cannot be shielded from the socially capricious milieu in which it is situated: 'Services for the mentally ill are in turmoil in many parts of Britain...with Government plans setting out how mental patients ought to be cared for...being widely ignored' (Fletcher 1995). The mayhem is signified through a never-ending deluge of policy initiatives, legislation, and recommendations from reports and inquiries.

In the last few decades in Britain, mental health practitioners and managers have been expected to: accommodate the independent sector; disentangle purchasers from providers, and health care from social care; introduce care plans for patients discharged from hospital; offer non-custodial care and treatment to mentally disordered offenders; reduce morbidity and suicide rates amongst the mentally ill; give priority to people placed on supervision registers; implement new mental health legislation; assess the risk of violence and homicide; replace care in the community with a 'spectrum' or 'continuum' of care; prepare for the possibility of an overarching planning and commissioning body; respond to the implications of the Patient's Charter; empower users and carers; audit clinical practice; reap the benefits of a succession of reviews concerning the education and roles of psychiatric nursing; assertively outreach; and comply with the outcomes of a reassessment of the whole of mental health law.

Furthermore, in the late 1990s the mental health services were invited to take on board the consequences of a critical dissection of the various professional groups by the Sainsbury Centre for Mental Health (1997). The comprehensive analysis of the work of mental health practitioners was a reaction to prolonged public concern about the competence of such groups as social workers, general practitioners, psychiatrists and psychiatric nurses.

Moreover, both health care workers and the public are exposed to political and/or media confusion over the future direction of care for the mentally disordered:

> A weekend report that care in the community was to be scrapped was repudiated by Frank Dobson, secretary of State for Health. [Dobson said] that there was a substantial minority of people who were either dangerous, or made such a nuisance of themselves that they needed 24-hour supervision – but that did not mean, as *The Daily Telegraph* reported [two days previously], that the entire care in the community scheme was to be abolished.
>
> (Bevens 1998)

Under the slogan of 'The Third Way', the Department of Health has launched its strategy to renovate all mental health provision. A cash injection of £700 million has been promised to accommodate a 'root and branch' overhaul of services. Furthermore, even though there have been centuries of state involvement in the management of madness, guidelines on 'national standards' will now be formulated (DOH 1998b, 1998c).

There is, therefore, much advice and many directives but little accord amongst politicians, the media and leaders of the mental health professions with regard to how society should deal with the mentally ill. What politicians, academics and leaders of such occupations as mental health nursing advocate today may not be the same as that which is promoted tomorrow.

Indeed, the contradictions and paradoxes of the postmodern era are conspicuous in one particular area of mental health policy. Whilst the rhetoric of 'empowerment' is directed enthusiastically towards the mentally ill, there are juxtapositional supplications about the threat of violence from those mentally ill people living in the community or about to be discharged from in-patient care (Morrall 1998a). That is, the policy of shifting power from the professions (and/or the state) to the users of the psychiatric services is at variance with the investment medicine and nursing have in retaining their relative and respective authority in society. It is also in tension with the social control function of psychiatric medicine and mental health nursing (Morrall 1998b).

Patterned chaos

There is a pattern within the chaos, however. Whatever social, political or economic discordance exists in Western society, the system remains remarkably stable, and unremittingly committed to a capitalist mode of production. Moreover, although there have been serious challenges to its dominance (for example, through the growth of 'complementary' medicine, and an increased interest in spirituality), scientific rationality persists as the core explanatory paradigm. Capitalism now has a global market, and techno-scientific discoveries (for example, transnational media networks) permeate virtually every culture in the world.

Furthermore, the ultimate function of psychiatry and psychiatric nursing, of operating on behalf of the state to prevent social ataxia, endures (Morrall 1998b). Medicine and nursing continue to monitor and regulate the form of deviancy (that is, 'madness') that is most challenging to capitalist rationalism. The pressure on the psychiatric professions to 'discipline' the non-conformist has increased not diminished.

The medical profession's formal powers to detain and/or forcibly administer treatment is still vigorous:

> A hospital...forcibly detained a sane woman in a psychiatric ward because she tried to starve herself to death...a former teacher and professional diver, suffered a series of strokes that left her unable to feed herself or to attend to her personal hygiene...Doctors wanted to administer electro-convulsive therapy (ECT) and forcibly re-hydrate her after she had stopped drinking.
> (Illman 1997)

As social control experts, psychiatrists are fundamental to the process of 'medicalising' a loose array and growing number of socially discordant behaviours (Scull 1993). In the fourth version of the American Psychiatric Association's (1994) manual of mental disorders there are eight hundred illness categories. These range from 'Alzheimer's Disease' to 'Female Sexual Arousal Disorder'!

However, psychiatry is relatively autonomous in its ability to operate as a profession and extend its practice without constantly reacting to the immediate exigencies of capitalist production. That is, psychiatry has been bestowed with the capacity to arbitrate, within a pre-set framework, the boundaries between normality and abnormality. It can also promote vested interests (as it did in gaining authority to manage the asylums). But this does not detract from the overall state-sanctioned task of psychiatry to oversee the socially unacceptable.

Nurses and social control

Psychiatric nursing is complicit in the enforcement of control in society. Nurses regulate behaviour, either indirectly (through their 'empathic' relationships with users of the mental health services) or directly (at the behest of psychiatrists or by their own actions). This becomes apparent when the mental health nurse is employed in the locked world of forensic psychiatry, whether this be in the special hospitals or secure units. It is obvious also when the nurse applies physical restraints to those in-patients whom are deemed to be 'uncooperative', or helps to maintain supervision registers for those living in the community.

Ironically, the intimate association that occurs between nurses and their clients in the institution or the community, whilst appearing magnanimous and serendipitous, can function as a covert, and therefore far more virulent, instrument of social control. In a study of twenty-eight nurses working in a general hospital setting, Sam Porter comments: 'Nurses' privileged position in their relationship with patients gives them plenty of scope to adopt strategies of inducement, encouragement or persuasion in order to influence the behaviour of patients' (Porter 1996: 74).

In the psychiatric setting (whether hospital or community) there is much more scope for the will of the nurse to preside over that of the client. The client is mentally distraught in one way or another and therefore *ipso facto* less likely to be effective in her or his assertions. Moreover, whilst indulging in humanistic and user-centred therapy (Dexter and Wash 1986), adopting a role as 'advocate' (Duxbury

1996), intervening as part of a 'Court Diversion Scheme' (Maclean 1995), or acting as 'liaison' to the police (Tendler 1995), nurses present as 'power-brokers', balancing the rights of the client with those of psychiatry and the state. However, in the final analysis, nurses are implicated in the process of dividing the sane from the insane, and/or the mad from the bad.

Aggregated disadvantage

For Scull (1979, 1983, 1984), psychiatry serves the capitalist state by keeping one section of the proletariat under control. Doctors and nurses serve as factotums of the state, assisting in the regulation of social deviance. The state in turn sustains the social system with all of its structured inequalities (for example, unemployment, homelessness, poverty, sexism, racism).

There is a strong correlation between psychiatric morbidity and social disadvantage (Rogers and Pilgrim 1996). The majority of users of the psychiatric services come from the lower end of the social hierarchy (Gallagher 1995). In my own study of 252 referrals sent to psychiatric nurses working in community mental health teams (Morrall 1995a, 1995b, 1997a, 1997b), the clients belonged to groups which are on the edge of mainstream society, and who suffer from substantial amounts of stigma. That is, most were unemployed, unpaid houseworkers, or retired. Moreover, most had received psychiatric care in the past, and over two-thirds would be retained within the psychiatric system.

Consequently, mentally disordered people endure an accumulation of disadvantage. For example, someone suffering from schizophrenia may also be homeless and poor. This leads to an amplification of her or his already 'spoiled' identity (Goffman 1963). She or he occupies the lowest rung in the hierarchy of social prestige, a segregated stratum even within the underclass.

Conclusion

Psychiatric doctors and nurses are implicated inexorably in the policing and exclusion of those on the perimeter of society. The *raison d'être* for both psychiatric medicine and nursing is the social control of the mentally disordered. This is a function of the state which is devolved to the psychiatric disciplines.

Traditionally, the asylum has been the architectural manifestation of the power of psychiatry. Non-institutional care has not expedited the predicted dissolution of psychiatry's rule as the pre-eminent profession in the field of mental health. Moreover, the fabric of Western society, whilst appearing ideologically, economically and socially to be disorganised and irresolute, remains relatively durable, and consigned to science and *logos*.

Furthermore, there are signs of a rebirth of asylumdom in the form of a projected growth in the number of 'secure units' in the community. Once again the asylum will symbolise emphatically the authority of the state (and its agencies of social control), and re-emphasise the exclusion of 'unreason' from 'reasonable' society.

References

American Psychiatric Association (1994) *Diagnostic and Statistical Manual of Mental Disorders*, 4th edition, Washington, DC: APA.

Audit Commission (1994) *Finding a Place: A Review of Mental Health Services for Adults*, London: HMSO.

Baruch, G. and Treacher, A. (1978) *Psychiatry Observed*, London: Routledge and Kegan Paul.

Bean, P. and Mounser, P. (1993) *Discharged from Mental Hospitals*, London: Macmillan/MIND.

Bennetto, J. (1998) 'Calls to check prisoners for mental illness', *The Independent*, 6 February.

Bevens, A. (1998) 'Dobson denies call to stop care in the community', *The Independent*, 19 January.

Blair, T. (1997) 'Why we must help those excluded from society', *The Independent*, 8 December.

Brooks, P. (1993) *Body Works: Objects of Desire in Modern Narrative*, Harvard: Harvard University Press.

Burgess, R.G. (1981) 'Keeping a research diary', *Cambridge Journal of Education*, 11, part 1: 75–83.

Burnard, P. (1991) 'A method of analysing interview scripts in qualitative research', *Nurse Education Today* 11, 461–6.

Carrier, J. and Tomlinson, D. (eds) (1996) *Asylum in the Community*, London: Routledge.

Cartwright, D. and Zander, A. (eds) (1968) *Group Dynamics*, 3rd edition, London: Tavistock.

Craig, T., Bayliss, E. Klein, O., Manning, P. and Reader, L. (1995) *The Homeless Mentally Ill Initiative: An Evaluation of Four Clinical Teams*, London: Department of Health/Mental Health Foundation.

Department of Health (DOH) (1998a) *The New National Health Service: Modern, Dependable*, London: Stationery Office.

——(1998b) 'Frank Dobson outlines Third Way for mental health', Press Release 98/311, 29 July.

——(1998c) 'Strategy launched to modernise the mental health service', Press Release 98/0580, 8 December.

Dexter, G. and Wash, M. (1986) *Psychiatric Nursing Skills: A Patient-centred Approach*, London: Croom Helm.

Dowding, K. (1996) *Power*, Buckingham: Open University Press.

Duxbury, J. (1996) 'The nurse's role as patient advocate for mentally ill people', *Nursing Standard* 10, 20: 36–9.

Fletcher, D. (1995) 'Care of mentally ill "in state of turmoil" ', *The Electronic Telegraph*, 25 August.

Foucault, M. (1971) *Madness and Civilisation*, London: Tavistock.

——(1973) *The Birth of the Clinic*, London: Tavistock.

Gallagher, B.J. (1995) *The Sociology of Mental Illness*, Englewood Cliffs, New Jersey: Prentice-Hall.

Goffman, E. (1963) *Stigma: Notes on the Management of Spoiled Identity*, Harmondsworth: Penguin.

Illman, J. (1997) 'Paralysed stroke victim who longed for death is forced into a psychiatric ward', *The Observer*, 23 March.

Johnson, S., Ramsay, R., Thornicroft, G., Brooks, L., Lelliott, P., Peck, E., Smith, H., Chisholm, D., Audini, B., Knapp, M. and Goldberg, D. (eds) (1997) *London's Mental Health: The Report to the King's Fund London Commission*, London: King's Fund.

Johnstone, L. (1989) *Users and Abusers of Psychiatry: A Critical Look at Traditional Psychiatric Practice*, London: Routledge.

Layder, D. (1994) *Understanding Social Theory*, London: Sage.

Lukes, S. (1974) *Power: A Radical View*, London: Macmillan.

Maclean, L. (1995) 'Community psychiatric nurses in relation to diversion schemes', in C. Brooker and E. White (eds) *Community Psychiatric Nursing: A Research Perspective*, Vol. III, London: Chapman & Hall.

Masson, J. (1992) *Against Therapy*, London: Fontana.

Mihill, C. (1995) 'Jobs denied to mentally ill', *The Guardian*, 1 September.

Morrall, P.A. (1987) 'Re-carceration: social factors influencing admission to psychiatric institutions, and the role of the community psychiatric nurse as agent of social control', *Community Psychiatric Nursing Journal* 7, 6: 25–32.

——(1995a) *The Professional Status of the Community Psychiatric Nurse*, PhD thesis. Loughborough: University of Loughborough.

——(1995b) 'Clinical autonomy and the community psychiatric nurse', *Mental Health Nursing* 15, 2: 16–19.

——(1997a) 'Lacking in rigour: a case-study of the professional practice of psychiatric nurses in four community mental health teams', *Journal of Mental Health* 6, 2: 173–9.

——(1997b) 'Professionalism and community psychiatric nursing', *Journal of Advanced Nursing*, 25, 1133–7.

——(1998a) 'Clinical sociology and empowerment', in P. Barker and B. Davidson (eds) *Psychiatric Nursing: Ethical Strife*, London: Arnold.

——(1998b) *Mental Health Nursing and Social Control*, London: Whurr.

Murphy, E. (1991) *After the Asylums*, London: Faber and Faber.

National Health Service Management Executive (1996) *Primary Care: The Future*, London: Department of Health.

Nolan, P. (1993) *A History of Mental Health Nursing*, London: Chapman & Hall.

Porter, R. (1987) *A Social History of Madness: Stories of the Insane*, London: Weidenfeld & Nicolson.

Porter, S. (1996) 'Contra-Foucault: soldiers, nurses and power', *Sociology* 30, 1: 59–78.

Poulantzas, N. (1978) *State, Power, Socialism*, London: New Left.

Rogers, A. and Pilgrim, D. (1996) *Mental Health Policy in Britain: A Critical Introduction*, Basingstoke: Macmillan.

Sainsbury Centre for Mental Health (1997) *Review of the Roles and Training of Mental Health Care Staff*, London: Sainsbury Centre.

Samson, C. (1995) 'The fracturing of medical dominance in British psychiatry', *Sociology of Health and Illness* 17, 2: 245–69.

Scull, A.T. (1979) *Museums of Madness: The Social Organisation of Insanity in Nineteenth Century England*, Harmondsworth: Penguin.

——(1981) 'Social history of psychiatry in the Victorian era', in A.T. Scull (ed.) *Madhouses, Mad-doctors and Madmen*, Philadelphia: University of Philadelphia Press.

——(1983) 'The asylum as community or the community as asylum: paradoxes and contradictions of mental health care', in P. Bean (ed.) *Mental Illness: Changes and Trends*, Chichester: Wiley.

——(1984) *Decarceration: Community Treatment and the Deviant – a Radical View*, 2nd edition, Cambridge: Polity Press.

——(1993) *The Most Solitary of Afflictions: Madness and Society in Britain, 1700–1900*, New Haven, CT: Yale University Press.

Smail, D. (1984) *Illusion and Reality: The Meaning of Anxiety*, London: Dent.

Tendler, S. (1995) 'Psychiatric nurse helps police to distinguish the mentally ill', *The Times*, 17 January.

Thompson, A. and Sylvester, R. (1998) 'Care in the community is scrapped', *The Daily Telegraph*, 17 January.

Timmins, N. (1996) 'GP reforms to revive cottage hospital care', *The Independent*, 11 June.

Turner, B.S. (1995) *Medical Power and Social Knowledge*, 2nd edition, London: Sage.

Unattributed editorial (1998) *The Guardian*, 13 January.

Waters, M. (1994) *Modern Sociological Theory*, London: Sage.

7 'You can go home today, Mrs Jones'

Surgeons' and patients' negotiations over discharge

Nick J. Fox

Introduction

Discharge from hospital marks the collision of two realms, that of the medical environment dominated by biomedicine, and a realm in which home, family and 'normal' life provide the primary textualities. The 'stripping' of identity (Goffman 1968) or, perhaps more accurately, the fabrication of an alternate identity as patient (De Swaan 1990) at the outset of a bout of hospitalization has been noted in the literature, but less attention has been paid to discharge from hospital. Decisions over discharge are considered in the medical literature to be primarily technical. However, just as other aspects of engagement between patients and health professionals are social activities (Fox 1993a, 1993b, Nettleton 1992, Roberts 1985, Silverman 1983), discharge from hospital takes place within a social context, and judgements by all concerned concerning discharge will never be free of 'social' components. As such, these judgements are tied up with the power and authority of those who make them, and decisions over discharge may be one way in which doctors sustain their control over interactions with patients. This chapter examines the micropolitics of interactions between patients and doctors around discharge following surgery. It explores the ways in which textualities deriving from different domains articulate to achieve discharge, and – by and large – to enhance and sustain medical definitions of situations.

The approach which has been adopted is post-structuralist and postmodern in provenance. Applied within social theory, post-structuralist epistemology contributes some new perspectives on agency and structure, continuity and change (Game 1991, Fox 1993a). In particular, it contributes an understanding of the relationship between 'power' and 'knowledge', of the part played by language and textuality in the fabrication of the world we inhabit and of subjectivity, and a recognition of difference and transformation as (dis)organising principles (in place of structure, continuity and similarity). The postmodern mood is more explicitly political, and the writings of Derrida, Lyotard and others are underpinned by political commitments to resistance and challenge to the 'victimization' of those who are the dispossessed (Derrida 1978: 28, Lyotard 1988: 13).

An influential strand in post-structuralism has been deconstruction, the approach developed by Derrida (1976) to explore the workings of power in the textual construction of the social world. Deconstruction has been applied in social theory to reveal the unspoken assumptions behind claims to 'truth' (Fox 1991, 1993a, Game 1991), and is of special use in exploring how particular discourses come to dominance, and what happens in situations where interpretations of reality are contested, for example by surgeons and anaesthetists (Fox 1994), or by teachers and child welfare professionals (Fox 1995a). The term 'deconstruction' has sometimes been used almost generically as a synonym for social analysis, but this is to dilute the methodology's focus on textuality and the strategies by which readings of situations are privileged both through and in the service of power. In general, it works by overturning these privileged readings, examining the way the world would look if the opposing view were to be dominant. As such, it is potentially both anti-authoritarian and a tool for resistance (Critchley 1992, Rosenau 1992).

In the coming pages I am going to develop a deconstructive strategy toward decisions to discharge patients following surgery, using three concepts from post-structuralism: Derrida's (1987) analysis of the *frame* or boundary as the place at which power acts; the general post-structuralist conception of *intertextuality* (Barthes 1977, Fox 1993a) and Lyotard's (1988) notion of the *differend*.

Texts, frames and *differends*

If a text is defined as any meaningful symbolic system, linguistic or otherwise, then intertextuality is the process whereby one text plays upon other texts (Barthes 1977). This play of text on text is endless – there can always be other points of reference for a text. At the simplest level, a dictionary definition refers to other textual elements (words), which in turn are defined by other elements. Similarly, this chapter makes reference to other texts, which in turn make other references, *ad infinitum*. The development of hypertextual and hypermedia software provides the technology for infinite intertextuality, in which not only books but films, music and other texts play in a limitless web (Landow 1992). Three propositions develop the relevance for social analysis of this notion of intertextuality.

1   In the study of the social, the primary unit of analysis is the *text*, which may be writing, bodily or social practice, or subjective sense-of-self, to which meaning may be ascribed. Texts are the product of human activity, and as such they are created within the flow of history, yet they are fragmentary, they are continually re-read and have no single or final meaning.

2   Texts engage with each other productively, and in this *intertextuality*, meaning comes into being, is sustained, distorted, obscured or reintroduced. The capacity to engage meaningfully with the social world – that is, to understand and to contribute to that world – is intertextual, a function of a subjectivity which is itself textual and not prior to textuality.

3   The 'meaning' of a text is thus not intrinsic. It can be understood as constructed where texts collide, or more specifically, in a text's *frame*, that is, at the boundary of that which distinguishes and bounds it from what it is not. Power is consequently a phenomenon of the *frame*: to write the limits of a text is a political act. But framing a text is always provisional, subject to challenge and renegotiation, and is always in the process of being achieved.[1]

There are a number of further implications which follow from these propositions, which are worth exploring before turning to the substantive data that will be subjected to this analysis. First, in intertextual approaches, the emphasis is upon the reader rather than the writer: a displacement of great significance for understanding power, knowledge and resistance. While texts are written by humans, their writers' *authorship* is provisional: authority is observable only at its site of action – that is, at the site of reading. Another way of putting this is to say that authority (the capacity to be acknowledged as 'speaking the truth') can never be possessed absolutely, it is always *achieved* and subject to resistance and challenge.

Second, intertextuality contributes endlessly not only to knowledge or 'ideology', but also to that special text which we call 'subjectivity' or sense-of-self. Using the notion of *framing* to explore this further, we come to see subjectivity as something dynamic, always in flux as intertextual readings contribute to a continuous process of *becoming-a-self*. Deleuze and Guattari (1984, 1988) describe this in their notion of a 'nomadic subjectivity', potentially free to wander through textuality, although always drawn to one framing (plateau) or another. In the data to be examined on discharge decisions, this is precisely what is happening, as the protagonists are framed as 'subjects' in one way or another.

But third, this is not to imply that an intertextual subjectivity is free to become whatever it may. In practice, framings are constrained in all sorts of ways. For Lyotard (1988), oppositional politics can be understood as a play of texts, what he calls 'phrases in dispute', all seeking to gain authority over the others. When one phrase gains ascendancy, it is by the denial of the intertextuality which might enable opposing discourses to 'prove' their own positions. As such, it becomes what Lyotard named 'the *differend*', a marker of the violence that is done in the name of discourse, the 'victimization' of other texts (1988: 9). A *differend* works by divesting others of the capacity to speak authoritatively or authentically; it is thus the constraining of intertextuality. Such constraint on intertextuality is necessarily imposed from outside of the discourse itself – by the threat of sanctions or through the use of other resources in the psychological or social world of the subject. Medical dominance, patriarchy, religious fundamentalism are all examples of *differends* – authentications of 'reality' which appear to be based on 'truth' because they deny alternative readings, and which are ultimately dependent upon the violence of technologies of power.[2]

In summary, the creation of a *differend* is an act of power which works at the margin or limit of a text. It frames that text (which may be a book or a social practice or a subjectivity), fabricating distance between author and object, self and other, what is and what is not. Deconstruction identifies these framings, exploring the achievement of *differends*. As a strategy, it upsets the accepted definitions, and looks not only at the content of a text (which is created only in relation to its framing), but through the positioning of the limits of text, how it is framed in relationship to that which is beyond. What is excluded is thus as important as what is included in a text or textual practice. Deconstruction reintroduces what has been left outside the frame.

Framing the text: decisions over discharge

Discharge following a period of hospitalisation is not, in law, a medical decision.[3] Any patient (other than those detained under mental health legislation) – if they are fit enough – may choose to discharge her/himself at any time. However, from the way in which discharge decisions are made, one might be led to believe that doctors are autocrats with absolute control over whether a patient stays in hospital or leaves. How is it that doctors can sustain this impression? Simplistically, one might argue that patients consign their autonomy to those who have responsibility for their care, acknowledging that specialist knowledge is sufficient warrant for this infringement of self-determination. But this assumes a consensual model of medical authority, and social scientists have argued that medical interactions must be understood as based on a variety of perspectives which vie for dominance (Strong 1978). So how exactly do doctors persuade patients to accept their version of reality over others?

This issue is of particular relevance following elective surgery. Consider the different phases of hospitalisation for such procedures. Before surgery, patients have chosen to come into hospital, and placed themselves under the authority of their surgeon. After the procedure has been carried out, and if the surgery is designated a 'success' by surgeon and other staff, the surgeon's version of reality is substantiated by the claims that the patient is 'cured' or ameliorated, in turn sustaining her/his authority to make such definitions. Yet the patient is often now demonstrably 'ill': the effects of surgery and anaesthesia having led elective patients to be considerably less well than upon admission (Fox 1994). This iatrogenic illness is acceptable up to a point, but the surgeon's authority is now open to challenge, because it is as a consequence of her/his actions that the patient remains in hospital, and the claims of the 'success' of the surgery are jeopardised by the continuing presence of the post-operative patient on the ward.

As time passes following surgery, the patient's condition usually improves and a surgeon is faced with a conflict, between discharging another 'success', and ensuring a patient is sufficiently recovered to be safely released from her/his gaze. And now the patient may seize on this conflict, to reassert her/his rights, to quit the uncomfortable environment of the hospital for home, family and 'normality'. The period leading up to discharge may thus be a time of difficult decisions, and of negotiation between doctor and patient, as the latter begin to redefine their situation within texts which are non-medical and relate to their biographical continuity. Surgeons face the possibility in such a situation that the definition of the situation will be inscribed in non-medical textualities, thereby losing their control both of the decision and, potentially, of their authority over it.

To examine the ways in which doctors negotiate this difficult time, I shall consider some data from my ethnographic study of surgery (Fox 1992). A number of post-operative ward rounds were observed on a general surgical ward and a gynaecology ward at two large teaching hospitals in the UK, and some of the interactions explicitly concerned discharge following surgery. The following analysis will not seek to achieve external validity or 'generalizability' (Lincoln and Guba 1985) through reports of a wide variety of encounters (from a post-structuralist position such claims of validity are merely rhetorical). Rather, three engagements where there is potential contestation of the decision to discharge will be explored using the perspective developed earlier. Each is relatively brief, but even so, they contain great richness in terms of the readings which the participants bring to the engagement.

Extract A: 'Fit or not fit?'

The first interaction occurred between surgeon Mr D and patient Mr Y during a post-operative ward round. The surgeon has a difficult decision to make, exemplifying the conflict of definitions of the patient as healed and yet iatrogenically 'ill'.

Mr D, the junior staff and the researcher gather round Patient Y's bed

Mr D: (*to patient, looking at chart*) Hallo, Mr Y. Well, we want to send you home, but I don't like that raised temperature.
Patient Y: No.
Mr D: I don't know what can be causing it. We've cultured the wound and there's no infection there. I just don't know what's causing it...Are things ready for you to go home?
Patient Y: Yes, my wife can come and collect me today.
Mr D: Can you go to bed, and she can look after you?
Patient Y: Yes.
Mr D: I don't like that raised temperature. Phone your wife and you can go home now.
Patient Y: Thank you very much.

It is worth beginning this first deconstruction by thinking about the textualities involved. The number of texts which might be discerned in this engagement is potentially endless (because of course, as readers we ourselves engage intertextually and thus productively with this text; see Fox 1995b), and there can be no 'final' or ultimately correct reading). But amongst others, we may identify: (a) The body of the patient, and the operation on Mr Y; (b) The context of the surgical ward; (c) Surgery as a discipline/skill/profession; (d) Mr D's professional occupation; (e) Mr Y's history as a patient, including the chart held by Mr D; and (f) Mr Y's biography, and his home and life outside the hospital.

Some of these are literally texts, while others are 'social' or 'body' texts, and the impact of each will depend on its framing. However, the deconstruction is not wholly unwieldy, as what are of interest are those frames which mediate the power relations of the encounter, in other words, those which serve as *differends*, violently disrupting the free flow of intertextuality, and working at a text's frame, at the delimitation of a text or where two or more texts collide.

What might be the *differends* here: the framings which write Mr Y and Mr D, silencing other voices, other textualities? There is the ward, and there is the bed which Mr Y is sitting upon, while Mr D and the rest of us stand over him. There is biomedicine, with its definitions and mystique of language. But perhaps the framing that is of greatest rhetorical use here is Mr Y's chart, on which is inscribed a text of his body in terms of temperature, heart rate, etc. The chart has a very literal frame, in that it covers the period of Mr Y's hospitalisation; beyond this temporal frame past and future cease to have any relevance. And it has a second metaphorical frame in its concerns with biomedically defined vital signs.

Mr D holds the chart, he is in control of it and Mr Y does not get to see it. Mr D uses the chart to frame the opening remarks, to mark out his authority over Mr Y's disposal. The chart frames Mr Y in terms of time and the signs recorded there. Nothing outside the frame of the chart is to be considered now, and the chart's biomedical framing sets the parameters within which the decision is to be made. Anything which is beyond the chart is excluded; Mr Y is written by the chart, he is the chart.

While this *differend* supplies Mr D's control of the situation, the framing is provisional, and Mr D admits this himself, because the chart reveals something disturbing about Mr Y: he has a raised temperature, a possible complication which will need to be resolved before discharge. Mr D 'doesn't like' this raised temperature. Why not? First, because it means Mr Y *is not fit*, not fit for discharge. Second (and he uses the identical phrase a second time), Mr D doesn't like it because it means Mr Y *does not fit* the framing which he wants to impose, of Mr Y as healed, an ex-patient, ready for discharge.

But Mr D wants this annoying temperature not to fit, to be excluded from his decision-making. So he must victimise it, creating a new *differend* to exclude it. Raised temperatures are things patients have, but Mr Y (Mr D wishes to demonstrate) is a non-patient, a success of surgery, he should have none of the attributes of a patient. To construct the *differend*, Mr D tests the limits of the text which is Mr Y and his raised temperature: the temperature is nothing to do with the operation ('there's no infection'), it is irrelevant ('I just don't know what's causing it'), Mr Y is ready to go home, his wife is ready to take him away, he will continue his recuperation at home, and he is physically capable of action ('phone your wife'). Mr D disallows the raised temperature any rights to define Mr Y. Mr Y is written as an ex-patient; no doubt in time, he will be written up.

Extract B: 'Stitched up'

In the second extract, discharge of Patient S is to be postponed, for a dramatic reason. Following an abdominal procedure, Mrs S's wound had burst. For surgeon Mr O, a 'success' of surgery, due to have been discharged, has been unexpectedly transformed into a 'complication' which is all too visible. For Mrs S, the expectation is now a longer stay in hospital.

Patient S is sitting in an armchair, looking very unhappy

Mr O: Hallo, Mrs S. Well, we were going to send you home yesterday, weren't we, and thank the God almighty we didn't.
Patient S: (*quietly*) No.
Mr O: Well, we just don't know why this happened, there's no infection, no haematoma, nothing at all to cause this. You were up and walking...?
Nurse: Yes she was walking about, and went to the lavatory and was straining, and then...
Mr O: ...Yes, I hear there was small intestine hanging out. Well, you've had a nasty time, and we'll keep you in for ten days.
Patient S: (*aghast*) Ten...days...?
Mr O: Yes, but there's absolutely nothing the matter inside, we don't know why this happened, so we'll keep you in for ten days.

Mr O had probably never expected to see Patient S as an in-patient again. She was out of the frame which she has occupied as a hospital patient, excluded and written down as a success of surgery. Now she is back again, and Mr O is faced with a difficult explanation, of why this success had so dramatically returned to haunt him. How could he have made what was effectively an incorrect decision to discharge this patient, whose very presence indicates she was insufficiently recovered to be sent home? Is he to blame for a framing which could potentially have had disastrous consequences had the wound burst once Mrs S had left hospital?

Mrs S's sutures supply Mr O with his *differend*, a new frame of reference which denies alternative readings and sustains his authority. What was inside has come out, it has burst through the stitches he put in place to frame Mrs S's success, and yet 'there's absolutely nothing the matter inside': Mr O cannot be held responsible; nothing he did – allowing infection or a blood vessel to leak – can be found to explain the burst sutures. Mrs S was showing all the signs of recovery, walking about the ward, using the lavatory. Now Mrs S has been stitched up again, what should be inside is back in place, and the wound sutures frame her surgery once again as a success – albeit one who has suffered complications.

In such circumstances, Mr O has little difficulty renegotiating a new discharge date, a very conservative distance ahead, so no new circumstance can challenge his authority to dispose of his patient appropriately. Mrs S is very much the victim of this *differend*, which denies any role for Mr O in this episode. Mrs S's exertions had caused her stitches to burst, now she must suffer the consequences. All that matters is that what is framed by the stitches remains so, Mrs S's biography is of no concern.

Extract C: 'I'll ask the questions'

Lyotard's analysis (1988) of the creation of *differends* emphasises the unequal nature of these power plays, dependent on all sorts of imbalances in resources between actors. Whereas Patient Y was compliant (perhaps because he was getting his desired discharge), and Patient S is literally and metaphorically stitched up. In the following extract, surgeon Mrs A has to work hard to sustain her authority against challenge, and it could be argued that she is left with little resource other than her role as the decision-maker. Mrs A had previously implied that Patient Z, an old lady whose recovery had been slower than expected after a major gynaecological procedure, might be discharged on the day this encounter took place.

Mrs A:	Hallo, Mrs Z, I think you can go home on Monday.
Patient Z:	On Monday, not today?
Mrs A:	No, I think we'll keep you in till Monday. (*to house officer*) Doctor, can you listen to her tummy...(*to patient*) Where do you live Mrs Z?
Patient Z:	In [name of district].
Mrs A:	On your own?
Patient Z:	Yes, but I've arranged for my sisters to come over to me...
Mrs A:	...Yes. (*to house officer*) Does that sound OK?
House Officer:	Yes, it's OK.
Patient Z:	They're nurses. They're not actually working any more, but they're qualified nurses...
Mrs A:	Yes, you can go on Monday. (*turns away and walks off*)

Surgeon Mrs A's opening gambit is immediately challenged by Patient Z, because it is at variance with a previous expectation. In response, Mrs A initiates a two-pronged interrogation. She asks the house officer to gather data for her to use within a textuality concerning recovery. He is told to listen to Mrs Z's abdominal sounds, and is then asked to confirm whether they are normal. However, the significance of this information is not passed back to Patient Z or discussed with the house officer. Simultaneously, the surgeon begins a search procedure concerning Mrs Z's situation as a potential ex-patient: where she lives, if she has carers. Mrs Z seizes on this to try to establish her own *differend* concerning the care she will receive at home, challenging Mrs A's assessment that she needs hospital care.

Mrs A is apparently left with few resources to sustain her authority. Neither line of questioning has provided data which supports the deferral of discharge. Even her question and answer strategy has been subverted by the patient's information about her carers. Yet she may resort to her status: she is the one standing up, who can walk away, leaving Mrs Z in bed; she is the one asking the questions and making the decisions. Mrs A ends by baldly re-stating her first utterance, and now it can be seen that her initial statement was intended to seize the initiative, to assert from the start her framing of herself as the decision-maker, and the patient as the fortunate recipient of this benign authority. In this situation, power validates itself, its victim remains a victim.

Final frame

Becoming a patient entails both a change of subjectivity (from person to patient), and entry into a status in which that subjectivity is influenced by medical authority, including the right to relinquish that subjectivity. Discharge from hospital is thus not simply a matter of physical displacement. Nor is it always merely the re-framing of subjectivity in some reflexive process of 'getting back to normal life'. The analysis which has been undertaken here suggests that the social processes involved in discharge are as much tied up with medical authority and power as any which take place between patients and health professionals. Surgeons use their authority to frame the subjectivity of their patients up to the moment of discharge, and where necessary do this through manipulations of texts which have been considered here as *differends*.

From an intertextual perspective, there is an infinite number of texts which may be written and read as we live out the social world. The undifferentiated events which make up the flow of history provide the raw material for this endless play of intertextuality. At the same time, 'history' (the texts we call the past and the present) is the product of intertextuality. Events, bodies and selves are written and read, as they are framed to provide meaningful textualities. Yet the number of texts which comprise the shared social world is often quite limited, there is not the massive proliferation of meaning which intertextuality implies.

In this study of the meanings surrounding the discharge of surgical patients, conflicting texts on the subjectivity of the patient (deriving from medical and biographical frames) come into play. In deconstruction, the 'inequality' between such texts becomes clearer, and we can begin to understand why some texts become dominant at the expense of others. First, the framing of texts which enables them to 'make sense' takes place in a context: the impinging universe of potential textualities, including the hospital's architecture and routines; the institution of biomedicine; the disciplines of medicine and nursing; and the biographical and medical history of the patient. Second, while new texts may be introduced to support one or another reading, the ability to introduce such texts depends on an environment which is supportive to 'other voices', and often, such an environment does not exist. Framing of texts sometimes leads to the creation of victims: those who are unable to speak in the face of a *differend*, a textual framing which violently refuses to permit of alternative readings.

Concerning discharge, we have seen this violence in action. Medical authority is the capacity to choose the framing of a patient's subjectivity, to include and exclude those texts which suit or do not, to serve the *differend* by which the patient is to be discharged or to remain a patient a little longer. Participants draw upon a variety of resources in these exchanges to support their claims to authenticity and authority: the discipline of biomedicine and the rights to self-determination of the human subject amongst others. When interpretations of events cease to be consensual, the achievement of outcomes depends on a naked exercising of power in the creation of *differends*.[4]

As a strategy, deconstruction is thus not only a methodology for qualitative data analysis, but a political tool which opposes authoritarian exercises of power in the denial of intertextuality. As such, this deconstruction of discharge decisions has clear political implications for 'patients' and health care 'professionals' over interactions over discharge, and at other points where subjectivities as patients and professionals are fabricated. The emphasis on violence and victimisation paints a less rosy picture of the way power works than those in traditional analyses of such 'negotiations'.

Deconstruction opens up the frame, questioning why some things are included and others excluded. Of course, at the same time, it creates its own framings, and any deconstruction can be subjected to similar interrogation itself. As such, deconstructive work is never final or complete: there is always another possible reading. Were this not the case, it would itself be a *differend*, violently refusing other voices. With this in mind, the strategy can supply the possibility of resistance, for new framings: of subjectivities which can 'become other', of voices which until now had been silent.

Acknowledgements

Thanks are due to the patients and surgeons at 'Western Hospital' who were participants in this study.

Notes

1 I am not here using the notion of a frame in the way developed in Goffman's (1974) *Frame Analysis*, in which a frame is to be understood as the sense-making definitions of situations, by which an individual

134   *Nick J. Fox*

comes to organise her experience (1974: 10–13). In this perspective, frames are phenomenological and are not concerned with social organisation or with social inequity (ibid.: 13–14). Building on Derrida's (1987) analysis of the frame as a boundary, I am arguing that framing *is* necessarily social, as the 'frame' of a text is the place at which power acts. Further, it is more than just the sense-making work of an individual, it can *be* that 'individual' inasmuch as it is at the frame of a text that subjectivity is fabricated. Readers might see some congruity between Goffman's *frame* (a set of organisational principles for making sense of experience) and *text* in my analysis, although I do not see such a comparison as useful. I reserve the term 'frame' for the limits of texts, where they are brought into opposition with other texts and thus engage with them in relations of power. It is this emphasis on the limit which is relevant in my own 'frame analysis'.

2   This position is congruent with Derrida's (1976) notion of *logocentrism*, the privileging of one version of the world such that it becomes possible for a speaker to be accredited with the capacity to speak the 'truth' (logos). However, readers will note that this position places greater emphasis on coercive power than Foucault's position, which considers disciplinary power to be typical of the modern period (Foucault 1980: 116–19). For Lyotard, while power may be mediated by knowledge, the right to claim 'knowledge' derives from the possession of power, and when the foundation of such knowledge is openly challenged, those in authority may exercise a more naked power, one which victimises and silences its opponent. Lyotard's version of power is much more negative than the 'creative' power of Foucault, which is often associated with post-structuralism.

3. Technically, a patient may discharge her/himself at any time 'against medical advice', in which case, the medical establishment is relieved of responsibility for a patient's well-being.

4   This is not to say that power is ever absolute: it is always possible to resist. 'Compliance' with medical advice is primarily an issue of authority, and refusal to comply marks a rejection of an ascribed subjectivity which confirms that authority. In this author's opinion, such a model of power has advantages over that espoused by Foucault because of its capacity to conceptualise possibilities for resistance. For a full discussion of this issue of resistance to power, see Fox 1993a, and for a comparison with Foucault's position, Fox 1997.

References

Barthes, R. (1977) *Image-Music-Text*, Glasgow: Collins.
Critchley, S. (1992) *The Ethics of Deconstruction*, Oxford: Blackwell.
Deleuze, G. and Guattari, F. (1984) *Anti-Oedipus: Capitalism and Schizophrenia*, London: Athlone.
——(1988) *A Thousand Plateaus*, London: Athlone.
Derrida, J. (1976) *Of Grammatology*, Baltimore: Johns Hopkins University Press.
——(1978) *Writing and Difference*, London: Routledge and Kegan Paul.

——(1987) *The Truth in Painting*, Chicago: University of Chicago Press.

De Swaan, A. (1990) *The Management of Normality*, London: Routledge.

Foucault, M. (1980) 'Truth and power', in C. Gordon (ed.) *Power/Knowledge*, Brighton: Harvester.

Fox, N.J. (1991) 'Postmodernism, rationality and the evaluation of health care', *Sociological Review* 39, 709–44.

——(1992) *The Social Meaning of Surgery*, Buckingham: Open University Press.

——(1993a) *Postmodernism, Sociology and Health*, Buckingham: Open University Press.

——(1993b) 'Discourse, organisation and the surgical ward round', *Sociology of Health and Illness* 15, 16–44.

——(1994) 'Anaesthetists, the discourse on patient fitness and the organisation of surgery', *Sociology of Health and Illness* 16, 1–18.

——(1995a) 'Postmodern perspectives on care: the vigil and the gift', *Critical Social Policy* 15, 107–25.

——(1995b) 'Intertextuality and the writing of social research', *Electronic Journal of Sociology* 1, 2: no page numbers. Available at http://www.sociology.org/vol001.002/fox.maintext.html.

——(1997) 'Is there life after Foucault? Texts, frames and differends', in A. Petersen and R. Bunton (eds) *Foucault, Health and Medicine*, London: Routledge.

Game, A. (1991) *Undoing the Social*, Buckingham: Open University Press.

Goffman, E. (1968) *Asylums*, Harmondsworth: Penguin.

——(1974) *Frame Analysis: An Essay on the Organization of Experience*, New York: Harper and Row.

Landow, G.P. (1992) *Hypertext*, Baltimore: Johns Hopkins University Press.

Lincoln, Y.S. and Guba, E.G. (1985) *Naturalistic Enquiry*, California: Sage.

Lyotard, J. (1988) *The Differend: Phrases in Dispute*, Minneapolis: University of Minnesota Press.

Nettleton, S. (1992) *Power, Pain and Dentistry*, Buckingham: Open University Press.

Roberts, H. (1985) *The Patient Patients*, London: Routledge and Kegan Paul.

Rosenau, P.M. (1992) *Postmodernism and the Social Sciences*, Princeton, NJ: Princeton University Press.

Silverman, D. (1983) 'The clinical subject: adolescents in a cleft palate clinic', *Sociology of Health and Illness*, 5, 253–74.

Strong, P. (1978) *The Ceremonial Order of the Clinic*, London: Routledge.

8 Empowerment and health

A community development approach to health promotion

Sue Davies

Introduction

A growing body of literature documents the detrimental effects that powerlessness can have on people's health. Traditional approaches to improving health have focused upon individual responsibility and/or behavioural techniques. However, these approaches largely ignore structural inequalities in health. Evidence is now accumulating to suggest that empowering communities to identify their own health needs and facilitating ways to address those needs can be a health-enhancing activity. This, however, may mean addressing problems not prioritised by professionals. Increasingly, as health professionals are required to achieve government-imposed targets in relation to specific health indicators, community concerns may be marginalised.

This chapter will describe a community development approach to promoting health through empowering communities and addressing issues of equity and access to health-enhancing activities. The background to the community health development movement will be outlined and the principles of this approach will be discussed. The chapter will then draw upon evidence from the evaluation of a community health development project in Beckton, East London, to highlight some of the benefits and challenges of this approach.

Excluded communities: a challenge for the millennium

The term social exclusion has been widely used to recognise not only the material deprivation of the poor, but also their inability fully to exercise their social and political rights as citizens (Geddes 1996). However, there is growing recognition that whole communities, as well as individuals, can experience disadvantage and exclusion

(Room 1995, Geddes 1996). New communities in particular may be affected by the disappearance of industrial employment, the breakdown of family structures and social isolation in neighbourhoods 'deserted by the middle classes' (Strobel 1996: 180). Certain social groups, such as members of ethnic minorities, lone parents and the unemployed, are more at risk of exclusion than others. Where these groups are over-represented within a community, then the whole community may be more vulnerable: 'where the material living standards and citizen rights of significant numbers of people are restricted by persistent multiple and concentrated deprivation, social cohesion may be threatened' (Geddes 1996: 10).

In some areas, urban regeneration has resulted in community exclusion as geographical boundaries have isolated families from their existing support networks. A focus on social housing projects within some programmes has resulted in an imbalance within the local population structure, with many of the groups at particular risk of social exclusion over-represented. When this is combined with the common feature of much urban renewal – that house-building is usually completed before the infrastructure and services are in place to support new residents – then the conditions for community exclusion are virtually complete.

The consequence for those living within excluded communities is that they become 'disempowered' by the structures which control and direct their lives, such as the benefits system, and housing and environmental policies. The effects include poverty, stress and communication and relationship difficulties, which in turn lead to a lack of self-confidence and self-esteem (Baker 1992). Such communities need to be empowered to take collective action, often by developing skills at an individual level to enable participation in the change process.

Approaches to health promotion and the rationale for the community development approach

Alongside the growing recognition of the detrimental effects of social exclusion on health, there appears to have been a 'revolution' in the field of health promotion during the past decade (see for example, Bernstein *et al.* 1994, Robertson and Minkler 1994). In particular, there has been a shift in emphasis from a focus upon individual behaviour change to more radical approaches which emphasise the need to change political and social structures. Similarly, empowerment approaches aimed at facilitating individual and community choices have gained in acceptance (Dines and Cribb 1993, Webb 1994, Airhihenbuwa 1994). This shift is reflected in position papers disseminated by the World Health Organisation (WHO), such as the Ottawa Charter (WHO 1986) and has been accompanied by widespread debate about what constitutes health and how health promotion should be organised and directed in order to be most effective.

Evidence in support of the empowerment approach to health promotion is accumulating. Research has focused upon the association between powerlessness and mental and physical health status (for example, Ryan 1967, Seligman 1975, Seeman and Seeman 1983, McKnight 1985, Braithwaite *et al.* 1989, Wallerstein 1992) and between stress and ill health (for example, House 1981, Cohen *et al.* 1986, Israel and Sharman 1990). On the basis of a review of this literature, Wallerstein concludes that, 'powerlessness can be thought of as a broad risk factor for disease and empowerment as a strategy for improving a population's health' (Wallerstein 1992: 204).

What is community health development?

Community health development has evolved from the notion of community development, which has been defined as 'a process whereby communities are empowered and enabled to express their health needs' (Smithies and Adams 1993: 58), and 'a way of working, informed by certain principles, which encourages people to identify common concerns and which supports them in taking action related to them' (Healthy Sheffield Support Team 1993).

The community development movement is underpinned by theories of human oppression, in particular the work of Paulo Freire (1972). Within the UK, interest in the concept of community participation in health and its association with community development has developed over the last fifteen to twenty years, largely in response to evidence of persisting social inequalities in health. A series of reports has recognised that the medical model approach to health promotion can do little to mitigate or prevent ill health associated with poverty (DHSS 1980, Whitehead 1987, BMA 1995). These reports identify a need for structural as well as individual approaches to health promotion in order to provide health services to meet health need. Concurrently, the need for community participation has received greater emphasis within WHO policy. The Alma Ata declaration in 1978 stated that: 'the people have a right and a duty to participate individually and collectively in the planning and implementation of their health care.' This idea was further endorsed by the WHO Targets for Health for All in 1985, which identified community participation as a basic tenet for the health-for-all philosophy.

These moves represent a major shift from the traditional reductionist biomedical model of health, disease avoidance and personal responsibility to a broader, more positive and holistic view of health and its determinants. However, the response from statutory services has been patchy. Some health authorities, and more recently community trusts, have appointed health promotion officers with a specific remit for community development. In some areas, health visitors have been encouraged to take on more public health responsibilities and to work in a different way with positive results (see, for example, Drennan 1988). However, on the whole, initiatives are characterised by poorly paid community workers on fixed-term contracts with inadequate funding, often working with little support and unrealistic objectives (Jones and Beattie 1991).

Community health development in Beckton

Beckton is a rapidly growing urban development on reclaimed land in East London, opposite Greenwich and south of East Ham. It has been described as sitting in the middle of a social and economic wilderness which has resulted from the decline of traditional Dockland industries. Together the London Borough of Newham and the London Docklands Development Corporation have developed a series of housing projects on this derelict land, which, although not envisaged as such initially, have developed mainly into social housing.

As with many new towns, development of the infrastructure to support the local community has not kept pace with housing development. There are major gaps in service provision: for example there is currently no secondary school within the area. The resident population is largely young and ethnically diverse, with many people dependent on state benefits. Housing is generally good and includes properties suitable for large families managed by housing associations. There are a number of potential employment opportunities, including the Millennium exhibition and a new university in the area. These initiatives reflect a growing sense of optimism for the future of Beckton.

When I first moved into Beckton, I moved from Forest Gate. It's a very busy area – lots of people, lots of things happening, all the shops. Then when I came to Beckton, all I saw was this new house, three bedrooms and yes I wanted it. Then, you know, live there and it was a bit of a shock. It was so quiet. I didn't know anybody cause you left all your friends – shops – where they are and all the handy things that you took for granted – they weren't in Beckton. So I found that a bit – oh dear, have I made the right choice – although I liked my house. I wasn't sure if it was the right place to be – I felt I was quite cut off from Newham. But over, say, the last six months, it's more people coming in, lots more places being built. It feels a bit better now.

(Local resident, recorded interview)

A small community development project funded by the local health promotion department had been set up at the St Mark's Church and Community Centre in Beckton in 1992. Funding for this work required that activities would aim to increase awareness of healthy eating and reduce smoking among the local population. However, the two workers involved soon recognised that these issues were not considered priorities by many residents, who expressed a need for initiatives to tackle wider issues, such as social isolation, racism and poverty. As a result, a more holistic approach to health promotion was adopted, resulting in local people identifying their own agendas and becoming equal partners in developing a diverse range of projects and community festivals.

The lack of published research exploring the effectiveness of the community development approach as a means of promoting good health contributed to the decision not to renew funding for this work. However, those who had been involved with the project believed there was a great deal of value in this way of working and began to look for further opportunities to develop such initiatives. There was also recognition of the need to reflect on methods used and to monitor and evaluate projects on a more systematic basis. This led to the development of a bid for funding for the establishment of a new project based upon similar principles and for a researcher whose role would be to focus on the effectiveness of the community health development approach. In May 1995, the King's Fund agreed to fund one full-time community health development worker for two years in the first instance, together with an evaluation of the project. A full-time project worker was duly appointed and commenced work in September 1995. The project worker was based at St Mark's

Church and Community Centre, a thriving organisation in the centre of Beckton, which provided a base for a number of community projects, including childrens' work, youth work, and activities for older people.

The Beckton Community Health Development Project: aims and objectives

The original stated aim of the project was to use a community development approach to promote well-being through reducing stress levels, depression and social isolation and to empower local communities to make healthy lifestyle choices for themselves and their children. The approach to community health development in Beckton was characterised by the following core values and principles:

- a commitment to tackle inequality and discrimination;
- a recognition of the need to give people more power over their lives and enable them to control the factors which affect their health and general well-being;
- a commitment to working with people, rather than for them;
- encouraging people to identify their own needs and agendas;
- recognising that many problems are interlinked;
- giving priority to activities relating to deprived groups and inequalities in health;
- recognising that the process of working together for health is as important as the outcomes.

Building upon previous work, the funded proposal identified three main objectives as follows:

1 To encourage local people to form common interest groups to help break down social isolation, reduce stress and depression and to increase confidence and develop social skills.
2 To develop an under-18s arts project, focusing upon improving the look of the local environment.
3 To work with local community workers to increase awareness of specific health issues with a focus on child health.

These principles and objectives provided the basis for developing the project in collaboration with local people and formed the focus of the evaluation.

Evaluation methodology

Much of the literature suggests that community development should be evaluated in stages (for example, Goodman *et al.* 1993). MacAllan and Narayan (1994) suggest that short-term evaluation could focus upon awareness of and participation in activities, medium-term could look at changes in knowledge, attitudes and behaviour, whereas long-term evaluation would need to consider changes in morbidity and mortality. Luck and Jesson (1996), reporting on the evaluation of the Corby CHOICE community development project, identify some practical objectives for evaluating community health development. These include whether the project has achieved predetermined objectives, survived and adapted to new circumstances and met the needs of different stakeholders. A recurrent theme within the literature is the need to look not only at outcomes but also at the process and elements necessary for achieving community empowerment. Process evaluation is essential in order to provide models for the design of future projects (Goodman *et al.* 1993).

On the basis of a review of more than forty reports of community health development initiatives, Alan Beattie (1991) has summarised the approaches to evaluation which have been adopted. Broad approaches include: action research, the project worker acting as evaluator; participatory methods involving project users; historical accounts and narratives and external evaluation. Methods include work diaries and work records, documentary methods, reports and minutes of meetings, memos and correspondence, participant observation, questionnaires, interviews, personal recollection moving towards oral history, group discussion, demographic and epidemiological statistics, naturalistic or ethnographic fieldwork, critical incidents and snapshots.

Beattie has categorised the range of approaches to evaluation and suggests that different strategies and methods appeal to the particular interests and concerns of different audiences and stakeholders. He suggests that the approach most in sympathy with the principles of community health development is the portfolio approach. This uses a mixture of data types and formats as a means of trying to make evaluation relevant to a variety of different audiences and interest groups.

Beattie suggests that the portfolio should constitute a cumulative, open-ended file of various types of information, qualitative and quantitative, representing the broad sweep of work in the project. The product is a resource which can be edited and put together in different formats for different audiences. This approach seemed appropriate for evaluating the Beckton project, since it has the potential to provide insight into the characteristics, processes and outcomes of community health development.

The evaluation funding was used partly to employ researchers on a consultancy basis to design and coordinate the evaluation in partnership with the Project Planning Team and local people. In order to reflect the community development approach, the evaluation aimed to use participative research methods as far as possible. As the programme of work developed, local people who had taken part in various aspects of the programme also became involved in collecting and analysing data for the evaluation. A combination of qualitative and quantitative methods was used, both to identify outcomes for the programme and to describe relevant features of its development and process.

The ultimate objective for the evaluation was to determine whether the Beckton Community Health Development Programme had achieved its stated aim of promoting the well-being of local people. Consequently, the evaluation attempted to answer the following questions:

1 What are the processes involved in establishing and developing a community development approach to health promotion?
2 Do local people perceive that they benefit from their involvement in projects initiated by the Community Health Development Programme and how do they benefit?
3 Does a community development approach to health promotion result in local people feeling more in control of their lives?
4 Does a community development approach to health promotion increase the potential for local people to make choices about their health-related behaviour?

Following Beattie (1991), the Project Team developed a pluralistic model of evaluation to ensure that the views and experiences of all groups of participants were reflected. Methods for evaluating the programme included:

• focused interviews with members of the Project Planning Team and project users at intervals in the development of the programme;
• maintenance of a tape-recorded reflective diary by the Community Health Development Worker;

- observation and process recording of key meetings of the Project Planning Team;
- video recording of selected project activities;
- semi-structured self-completion questionnaires to local workers in both statutory and voluntary agencies to record perceptions and experiences of the development of the programme and its effects;
- written statements by local people who had had close involvement with the project about their perceptions and experiences.

Main findings: events, processes, experiences, outcomes

For the purposes of this chapter, the main findings of the evaluation will be summarised in three sections. In order to illuminate the process of community health development (CHD), the main phases in developing the project are outlined. Specific activities which reflect the nature of the approach used are then presented, drawing upon the full range of information contributing to the evaluation. Key issues for the future development of CHD projects are then discussed.

Four overlapping stages were discernible in the development of the project:

1   Getting to know you – networking and developing relationships, both with local people and local workers.
2   Developing ideas – identifying priorities and making plans.
3   Making things happen – motivating, initiating, supporting and recognising when to withdraw.
4   Reflecting for the future – evaluating what has been achieved and developing proposals for extending the project.

During the first eighteen months, the project worker became involved in a wide range of events and activities (listed below). Those asterisked were established as a direct consequence of the project; those in italicised bold are described as case studies within this chapter:

- Asian Women's group*
- Women's group
- Carer and toddler group
- *Peer education group* (young people)*
- St Mark's playgroup
- Motorcycle group*

- Disabled anglers association
- *The Fantastic Seven* (Health needs assessment survey)*
- Parent in action group*
- Ladybirds (new parents group)
- Sexual health day*
- *Floating sculpture* (week-long arts event)*
- Mosaic mural (currently at planning stage)*
- Garden project (currently at planning stage)*

The number of groups and activities established in a relatively short space of time is testament to the success of the project in identifying needs and encouraging people to form common interest groups. Interviews with users of the project suggest that such initiatives achieved the objective of reducing social isolation for some people.

Outcomes identified by local people for the range of project activities included:

- increased self-confidence and assertiveness;
- increased use of local facilities and participation in events;
- reduced social isolation;
- changes in knowledge;
- changes in attitudes (HIV and AIDS, sexual behaviour, gender issues, racism);
- changes in behaviour (drugs, smoking).

A few key events and initiatives particularly reflected the principles of community health development and illustrate how these outcomes were achieved. These are presented here as brief case studies and illustrated with extracts from the evaluation data.

Peer education group

The peer education group developed from a need to engage young people in activities which would foster a sense of ownership and belonging within St Mark's and which would consequently reduce disruptive behaviour within the centre. Concurrently, the baseline interviews had suggested a need to raise young people's awareness of a number of health issues, such as drugs and safe sex. The project worker had already spent some time on the streets with local youth workers as part of her initial orientation. When one of the youth work leaders brought the issue of young people's disruptive behaviour to a staff meeting and asked for support, the project worker offered to organise some sort of activity. The staff team agreed that a trial period of a discussion-based group would be appropriate. This idea was introduced by the project worker to young people 'hanging around' the foyer of the building. As she describes it, she 'created a dialogue as young people came into the building and got their names right'.

The discussion sessions started with a group of three, but the numbers quickly swelled, and young people started to attend from outside the area. Some sessions were attended by up to twenty young people. 'Word got round that there was this mad black woman at St Mark's.' The young people themselves were encouraged to decide when they wanted to have a session. They also decided the focus for discussion, which was often something current within the media. Topics covered during the first series of sessions included sexual health and assertiveness, masturbation, drugs, religion, BSE, animal rights and racism.

At each session, ground-rules were established in relation to issues such as confidentiality and managing interruptions. Most sessions lasted two hours. During discussion, the project worker used a facilitative rather than educative approach, illustrated by the following extract from the transcript of one session when the focus was on drugs:

A: Do you take E's still now?
B: Sometimes, I should have done one on Saturday, but then I thought no.
C: I'd do a trip as well.
B: When I thought about it I thought no.
A: Why?
B: I don't know.
A: There must be some reason.
B: [Name] in the pub, he was saying do it and I thought no.
A: Is it because of Leah Betts?
B: It did influence me a bit.

It was apparent from entries in the project worker's reflective diary that sometimes the discussion challenged her own views and beliefs:

We were discussing about the beef, about the Mad Cow's Disease. It was a real uncanny session because, I suppose looking on my own perception as an outside member of the group, not thinking they had any compassion for animals or the welfare of animals and in this particular group a majority of the boys who are normally Mickey taking or disruptive were very serious in their dialogue in reference to animals and Mad Cow's Disease, initially it came up about foxes, one of the boys was quite pertinent about why are you killing animals and not killing people who are killing people, he was quite aggressive and assertive about that. His belief in saving animals was overwhelming and further on into the session he was backed by a few other what I would call rowdy boys.

The potential value of the group in bringing young people together in a safe environment to challenge and educate each other is also illustrated by an extract from the same diary entry:

> In terms of the Mad Cow's Disease it was the feeling of how long's this been going on? Was this going on before we were even born, there was some scepticism around the whole issue of the government, the Mad Cow's Disease and human behaviour. The group were quite perceptive about where they lie in society and it feels like unless you do get a group of young people into a room it's quite easy for them to be in society and be quite isolated and I suppose that I may have seen this a long time ago but I believe it was just more coherent for me then and believing that young people are well aware of what's going on around them and how the media and the news explain things.

The young people's written evaluations of the sessions were very positive:

> Normally I would go to Beckton Youth Project to do activities, but sitting and just talking with other kids, and knowing that it is confidential, and you can say what you want within reason is good. Sharon makes sure that everyone gets a chance to share their views, and experiences and opinions.

> Guess what? I never really knew that 'T' felt that way about animals, and I learned a lot from him tonight.

A specific need highlighted in the Young Peoples' Peer Education Group led to the development of a four-week programme on domestic abuse in association with Newham Action Against Domestic Violence. The group looked at relationships and at different types of abuse, including verbal, emotional and physical abuse. The programme involved smaller group exercises, discussions and opportunities for self-evaluation and exploring attitudes and values in a safe environment. The series ended with a drama production in which the young people acted out a situation in the form of a role play, with young men playing the part of women. This was recorded on video:

> I thought domestic violence was physical, it's about hitting. But when I call her a name I didn't see it as being classed as abuse – I didn't believe my words could have that much power.

> I've learned about emotional abuse – sending to Coventry is not a good way to sort out arguments.

> Doing the video was good – I felt the fear that the woman would feel when I played her – even my body language showed this in my role on the video which I didn't realise I'd done till we all saw the film.

Floating sculptures

This was a week-long arts event which was initiated when it became apparent that other events aimed at the second project objective of establishing an under-18s arts project, such as the mosaic mural, were going to take a while to set up. The floating sculptures were planned to happen fairly quickly and spontaneously. The event was coordinated by the project worker in liaison with Beckton Youth Project, the local neighbourhood worker, a local theatre group, the park rangers and the Borough Leisure Services. The aims of the event were to promote health through play and creativity, and to promote the Beckton Adventure Playground – a new initiative in the area. A five-day art workshop culminated in the launch of the floating sculptures on the lake in Beckton Park and a barbecue. Over forty young people, aged between nine and sixteen, together with some parents attended the workshop and launch. The project gave participants the opportunity to be involved in designing, making and exhibiting a large imaginative sculpture, which made a powerful environmental impact on a familiar setting: 'It achieved some sort of community coming together...on that day the sub-groups were eradicated and they became one group. Everyone was working together as a collective.'

As with most events within the Community Health Development Programme, the floating sculptures enabled the project worker to make contact with people not normally involved with St Mark's who have since become regular users. It also gave people the opportunity to socialise: 'It helped people to get to know each other which was what I was looking for...people to interact together where they weren't doing it before.' It was also fun:

> the second the bouncy castle went up the heavens opened...it was this freak weather...and there was Nick and Sharon – you couldn't see their faces for hail stones and they got a pedal boat because all the floating sculptures had turned upside down so they went out on a pedal boat with an umbrella just to rescue these sculptures. It was really funny!

Health needs assessment: The Fantastic Seven

Early meetings of the Project Planning Team identified a need to involve as many local people as possible in determining the focus of the programme. It was decided that a questionnaire survey was the most appropriate way to do this, and a small project group of volunteers (*The Fantastic Seven*) was established to take this work forward. *The Fantastic Seven* were all young women with children who lived locally, none of whom had any previous experience of developing a questionnaire or carrying out a survey. The group met on seven occasions to draw up the questionnaire and decide how to administer the survey.

The team decided to send the questionnaire to every household in the area and felt that the most cost-effective way to do this was to include it with one of the free newspapers delivered locally. Five thousand copies of the questionnaire were printed, and approximately 4000 were delivered. The team reached a consensus as to the area which they felt constituted 'Beckton'. Unfortunately, at the last minute plans to have the questionnaire delivered with the local newspaper fell through, and so local young people were recruited to deliver the questionnaire to every household, and paid from the evaluation budget.

In an attempt to improve the response rate, the opportunity to take part in a prize draw was offered to all who returned completed questionnaires. Prizes were donated by local organisations. In spite of these efforts, the initial response to the survey was very disappointing, with only 150 questionnaires received by the date for return.

Somewhat disheartened, the project team arranged for volunteers to complete questionnaires face-to-face with people in the street, and this approach swelled the number of respondents to 239.

Meetings of *The Fantastic Seven* were lively and generated a great deal of discussion and debate. In particular, transcripts of project meetings show how involvement in the survey challenged the views and attitudes of some group members. This is reflected in an extract from one of the interviews:

> I've made certain observations along the way. It got deeper than I thought it would do. A classic example is...we had decided as a group that we didn't want the ethnic box on the questionnaire but it was brought up at the Steering Group that perhaps it should be in there. So we went away and we met again...There was S, V, Myself, J and K discussing why we should or shouldn't have this box. I was quite positive that I didn't want this box – I couldn't see it would serve any purpose. I sort of talked everybody round and I convinced them that we didn't need this ethnic box. Then I thought – there are four white people here and two black – we are the majority so perhaps I'm wrong. It did make me think that everything I'd said was a particularly white thing and that made me look in another direction.

The project researcher set up a database and taught one of the project users how to code and enter the data on to computer. This person then took responsibility for coding, entering and cleaning the data: 'It's been a real eye-opener – some of the responses are really sad.'

At the time of writing, the project team were planning to feed back and validate the findings of the survey at a day-long workshop. This event will also generate ideas for using the findings to guide the work of the project.

Meeting objectives

In considering the extent to which the project was successful in meeting its objectives during the first eighteen months, it would appear that the emphasis was mainly on the first objective of encouraging local people to form common interest groups. This seemed appropriate, given the need to establish contacts and relationships in order to identify needs and plan activities to meet those needs. At time of writing, the project is at the stage of developing an extended programme of activities in order to engage with a wider range of groups within the local community and build upon the foundations of the first year's work.

An important objective of the Community Health Development Project was to bring about an increased level of involvement and inter-agency working between health workers in the statutory and voluntary sectors. This met with varying degrees of success and, although the project worker collaborated with the health promotion department on several successful initiatives, it proved more difficult than anticipated to engage other health service employees in the activities of the project. In spite of expressed enthusiasm for the community health development approach, attendance at meetings and events by workers such as community nurses and GPs was extremely limited. Contact with health workers suggested that this was due to overwhelming workloads rather than a reluctance to get involved. However, this unexpected difficulty suggests that the approach to working with health professionals needs to be revised. One idea is to establish a Health Forum to look at specific issues (domestic violence, for example) and invite all interested workers to attend. Anecdotal information suggests that other areas have had some success with this focused approach.

Contact and collaboration with workers in the voluntary sector was good, and the project also engaged with a range of local authority personnel, including environmental officers, social services staff and neighbourhood workers. Collaboration involved activities relating to child health – initiating first aid classes for members of the carer and toddler group, for example.

Key issues for future projects

A number of issues emerged during the course of the evaluation which might help to guide others in using a community health development approach. Themes emerged during the analysis of interview transcripts, diary entries and transcripts of meetings which were entered into a matrix and cross-referenced across data sources. Given the limited information available to describe the process of community health development generally, in particular the challenges likely to be faced by anyone using this approach, these issues are now described.

The importance of an established base

Compared with other projects which have started from scratch in setting up a base, the Beckton project had an important advantage in that it was based at an established centre with a range of activities already in progress. Hence the project worker had something to offer when she first made contact with people. Certainly many people became regular users of St Mark's after their first encounter with the project.

> That's how we came down here (Parent in Action group). Sharon got us a room, we sat down and discussed what we had to discuss and that was it. Ever since then I've been totally committed to St Mark's....I don't think other people in the community actually know what goes on here.

However, becoming a member of an established staff team also raised a number of difficulties for the project worker. In particular, it was difficult to maintain an appropriate balance between getting involved in existing activities and setting up new initiatives more in line with the project objectives. At times, the project worker found herself managing the crèche, for example, simply because there was no one else available within the building. In general, these distractions from the work of the project happened only in urgent situations. The issue was recognised early on by the project team, but the balance between being a member of the team and working to the project objectives has continued to provide a challenge.

Managing relationships

As with other projects, this evaluation has demonstrated the importance of strong relationships and effective dialogue to the success of community health development. Making people feel valued and encouraging them to feel that they have a role to play are fundamental to the principles of this approach. The skills of the project worker in making contact with people, informing them about the project and judging when they were ready to become involved were felt to be a major factor in establishing so many activities and events within a short space of time.

However, when people are working so closely together there is a danger of dependency. With a fixed-term project, there is also the potential problem of leaving people unsupported when funding runs out. The project worker was well aware of these dangers and the need to encourage users of the project to develop a network of contacts and relationships. Indeed, by the interim report stage there were signs that this was beginning to happen.

Getting people involved

Although most of the events and activities initiated within the Community Health Development Project were well supported by local people, it proved a continuing challenge to widen the circle of people involved. In particular, it proved difficult to maintain input from local people to the Project Planning Team. Interviews with project users suggested that some found the meetings quite daunting and didn't feel clear about their role. In these circumstances they found it difficult to contribute to discussion. This is likely to be an ongoing challenge for projects of this kind, since the balance between avoiding patronising people and creating the conditions in which they feel able to participate is difficult to achieve. A related issue is the need to ensure that any output from the project in the form of reports and write-ups needs to be accessible to as many people as possible.

The poor response to the health needs assessment survey also illustrates the difficulty of ensuring that everyone's voice is heard and that priorities for community health development projects are not determined by the views of a vocal minority.

A further example of the difficulty of motivating people to take part in community activities arose from concern about overhead pylons in Beckton. This has been an ongoing environmental issue in Beckton, with repeated calls for the power companies involved to relocate the electricity supply lines underground. The issue was resurrected during the course of the project, when two children attending the same school in Beckton developed leukaemia. Power cables run directly over the playground of the school concerned.

A public meeting organised by the local authority and attended by forty local residents provoked heated and acrimonious debate. However, attempts by the project worker and a local neighbourhood worker to establish an environmental issues group to coordinate the activities of local residents in relation to these perceived effects to health met with a resounding lack of response. This is further evidence of the need to create the conditions which allow those who are amongst the poorest and the most marginalised in society to participate in community action. Further work is required to establish what these conditions might be.

Keeping people involved

With some activities, it proved difficult to sustain momentum, in spite of initial enthusiasm. An example was the health needs assessment where, for a variety of reasons, the members of the original project group who designed the questionnaire were not available to be involved in the analysis. It was possible to involve new local people in this phase, but it is likely that the original group would have gained much more from the experience if they had been able to be involved in all stages of the survey.

A possible contributory factor may have been the timescale for preparing and administering the health needs assessment. Several people mentioned that it seemed to have taken a very long time to get the questionnaire ready (six months altogether). This may be a consequence of having one worker who is involved in a number of activities concurrently. However, several studies have identified the importance of providing immediate feedback to local people on the effects of community health development initiatives (Goodman *et al.* 1993). Consequently, it seems important to ensure that activities are completed within an appropriate timescale and not allowed to 'drag on' unnecessarily. The contribution of a structured programme built around clear objectives with predetermined deadlines is likely to be significant. This issue also highlights the importance of effective and regular supervision for those in a community health development role.

Models for community health development

The project presented an enormous challenge for one worker, and at times the project worker seemed quite isolated. The project team developed a number of bids for additional funding to support a second worker, but none was successful. Funding for two workers would have allowed the selection of applicants with complementary skills and experience and facilitated the provision of mutual support. Titchen and Binnie (1993) describe a collaborative partnership approach to action research in which one partner acts as the main initiator and the other as the main evaluator of an innovation. Within this broad role definition, there is role overlap and collaboration between the two partners This would seem to be an ideal model for community health development, given the lack of knowledge about this approach and the importance of systematic evaluation as part of any new initiative.

Conclusion

Although some of the events and activities initiated by the Beckton Community Health Development Project do not appear to have an overt health focus, the commitment to encouraging local people to identify their own needs is fully in line with the principles of community health development. The evaluation provided evidence that enabling local people to recognise that they can take control over even small aspects of their day-to-day lives resulted in increased confidence and well-being, and this was reflected in the findings of the interim evaluation report. The outcome for the Project Team was that the Kings Fund renewed funding for a further three-year period.

It would appear from this preliminary evaluation that community health development has the potential to break down some of the isolation and powerlessness resulting from community exclusion, significantly improving the sense of well-being for individuals. A longer-term evaluation will provide further insights into the processes and outcomes of this approach.

Acknowledgements

I would like to thank all members of the Project Team and the people of Beckton who contributed to the activities on which this chapter is based.

References

Airhihenbuwa, C.O. (1994) 'Health promotion and the discourse on culture: implications for empowerment', *Health Education Quarterly* 21, 3: 345–54.

Baker, J. (1992) *Family Health and Community Project Information Pack*, Family Health and Community Project, Newcastle-upon-Tyne: Cowgate.

Beattie, A. (1991) 'The evaluation of community development initiatives in health promotion: a review of current strategies', in J. Jones and A. Beattie (eds) *Community Development and Health Education*, Health Education Unit Occasional Papers, Vol. I, Milton Keynes: Open University Press.

Bernstein, E., Wallerstein, N., Braithwaite, R., Gutierrez, L., Labonte, R. and Zimmerman, M. (1994) 'Empowerment Forum: a dialogue between guest editorial board members', *Health Education Quarterly* 21, 3: 281–94.

Braithwaite, R., Murphy, F., Lythcott, N. and Blumenthal, D. (1989) 'Community organisation and development for health promotion within an urban black community: a conceptual model', *Health Education* 20, 5: 55–60.

British Medical Association (BMA) (1995) *Inequalities in Health*, London: British Medical Association.

Cohen, S., Evans, G., Stokols, D. and Krantz, D. (eds) (1986) *Behaviour, Health and Environmental Stress*, New York: Plenum.

Department of Health and Social Security (DHSS) (1980) *Inequalities in Health: Report of a Research Working Group* (Chair: Sir Douglas Black), London: HMSO.

Dines, A. and Cribb, A. (1993) *Health Promotion: Concepts and Practice*, Oxford: Blackwell Scientific.

Drennan, V. (1988) *Health Visitors and Groups: Politics and Practice*, Oxford: Heinemann Nursing.

Freeman, R., Gillam, S., Shearin, C. and Pratt, J. (1997) *Community Development and Involvement in Primary Care: A Guide to Involving the Community in COPC*, London: King's Fund.

Freire, P. (1972) *Pedagogy of the Oppressed*, Harmondsworth: Penguin.

Geddes, M. (1996) *Partnership against Poverty and Exclusion: Local Regeneration Strategies and Excluded Communities in the UK*, Bristol: The Policy Press.

Goodman, R.M., Steckler, A., Hoover, S. and Schwartz, R. (1993) 'A critique of contemporary community health promotion approaches: based on a qualitative review of six programs in Maine', *American Journal of Health Promotion* 7, 3: 208–20.

Healthy Sheffield Support Team (1993) *Community Development and Health: The Way Forward in Sheffield*, Sheffield: Healthy Sheffield Support Team.

House, J.S. (1981) *Work, Stress and Social Support*, Reading, MA: Addison-Wesley.

Israel, B.A., Checkoway, B., Schulz, A. and Zimmerman, M. (1994) 'Health education and community empowerment: conceptualising and measuring perceptions of individual, organisational and community control', *Health Education Quarterly* 21, 2: 149–70.

Israel, B.A. and Sharman, S.J. (1990) 'Social support, control and the stress process', in K. Glanz, F. Lewis and B. Rimer (eds) *Health Behavior and Health Education: Theory, Research and Practice*, San Francisco, CA: Jossey-Bass.

Jones, J. and Beattie, A. (1991) *Community Development and Health Education*, Health Education Unit Occasional Papers, Vol. I, Milton Keynes: Open University Press.

Luck, M. and Jesson, J. (1996) *Evaluation of Community Health Development*, Bath: Community Health UK.

MacAllan, L. and Narayan, V. (1994) 'Keeping the heart beat in Grampian: a case study in community participation and ownership', *Health Promotion International* 9, 1: 13–20.

McKnight, J.L. (1985) 'Health and empowerment', *Canadian Journal of Public Health* 76, 37–8.

Robertson, A. and Minkler, M. (1994) 'New health promotion movement: a critical examination', *Health Education Quarterly* 21, 3: 295–312.

Robottom, I. and Colquhoun, D. (1992) 'Participatory research, environmental health education and the politics of method', *Health Education Research* 7, 4: 457–69.

Room, G. (1995) *Beyond the Threshold: The Measurement and Analysis of Social Exclusion*, Bristol: Policy Press.

Ryan, W. (1967) 'Preventive services in the social context: power, pathology and prevention', in B. Bloom and D. Duck (eds) *Preventive Services in Mental Health Programs*, Boulder, CO: Western Interstate Commission for Higher Education.

Seeman, M. and Seeman, T.E. (1983) 'Health behaviour and personal autonomy: a longitudinal study of the sense of control in illness', *Journal of Health and Social Behaviour* 24, 144–60.

Seligman, M. (1975) *Helplessness*, San Francisco, CA: Freeman.

Shor, I. and Freire, P. (1987) *A Pedagogy for Liberation*, South Hadley, MA: Begin and Garvey.

Smithies, J. and Adams, L. (1993) 'Walking the tightrope: issues in evaluation and community participation for Health for All', in J. Davies and M. Kelly (eds) *Healthy Cities: Research and Practice*, London: Routledge.

Strobel, P. (1996) 'From poverty to exclusion: a wage-earning society or a society of human rights?', *International Social Science Journal* 48, 173–89.

Titchen, A. and Binnie, A. (1993) 'Research partnerships: collaborative action research in nursing', *Journal of Advanced Nursing* 18, 6: 858–65.

Wallerstein, N. (1992) 'Powerlessness, empowerment and health: implications for health promotion programs', *American Journal of Health Promotion* 6, 3: 197–205.

Webb, P. (1994) *Health Promotion and Patient Education: A Professional's Guide*, London: Chapman and Hall.

Whitehead, M. (1987) *The Health Divide – Inequalities in Health*, London: Health Education Authority.

World Health Organisation (WHO) (1986) *Ottawa Charter for Health Promotion*, Copenhagen: World Health Organisation.

Zimmerman, M. and Rappaport, J. (1988) 'Citizen participation, perceived control, and psychological empowerment', *American Journal of Community Psychology* 16, 5: 725–50.

9 Older people and health services
The challenge of empowerment

Alan Walker

The main purpose of this chapter is to examine the role of health services in creating and reinforcing exclusion among older people. It begins with an analysis of the role of professionals in constructing dependency in old age and the impact of age discrimination. This is followed by a brief discussion of the ways in which the imposition of market principles in health and social care in the 1980s reinforced the exclusion of older people. Finally attention is focused on overcoming the barriers to the inclusion of older people as active participants in decisions concerning their own health and social care, and some basic 'principles' of empowerment are proposed to assist the process of giving a voice to frail and vulnerable older service users. Throughout this discussion references to 'services' includes both health and social care because both occupy important roles in the lives of frail older people and because the boundary between them is often difficult to draw.

Professional power and the construction of dependency

Traditionally the sociological analysis of professions has tended to emphasise a hierarchy with, of course, medicine at the top, and below that profession are subordinate layers (sometimes labelled para-professions) including nursing and social work, followed by physiotherapy, chiropody, occupational therapy, and so on. Then there are occupations which are not usually described as professions but which sometimes aspire to a similar status to the occupations above them – home helps, home care assistants and residential workers. The main 'users' (or clients/patients) of the health and social care services are older people, therefore professional and para-professional groups in these services have a particularly important influence on the care and well-being of older people. Moreover, as is argued below, they have a crucial role as agents or gatekeepers with regard to the inclusion or exclusion of older people in the health and social services.

Ever since the advent of the welfare state, there has been a complex relationship between professionals and older people. As far as professionals are concerned, the formative years of all European welfare states were associated with a highly optimistic perception of their role. Indeed, some politicians regarded the expansion of the health and social care services as being synonymous with the production of welfare – the one automatically led to the other. By the 1970s, however, critical analyses of the role of professions had begun to point to various problems – such as the exercise of professional power in self-interested ways, particularly by the medical profession (Freidson 1970a, 1970b, Wilding 1982). Older people, despite their numerical importance, were often the least favoured by the high-status professionals. Thus, paradoxically, it was those at the bottom of the traditional professional hierarchy that were and still are mainly responsible for the largest client group of the welfare services.

At the same time, in social gerontology, a new strand of analysis was emerging which cast the welfare state and its professionals in a much less optimistic light than previous theories. This focused on what is called the social construction of dependency in old age (Walker 1980, 1982) which, with other contemporary work, produced the political economy of ageing paradigm (Estes 1979, Guillemard 1980, Phillipson 1982, Townsend 1981). This paradigm adopted a different perspective from the traditional social policy and gerontological approaches, which saw older people as a distinct social and biological minority, in isolation from social processes and values. It argued that the social and economic status of older people is defined not by biological age but by the institutions organised wholly or partly on production, especially the labour market, and by those institutions designed to administer or 'bureaucratise' old age, particularly the welfare state. Social policies are seen, therefore, as part of the process of defining old age in different societies, and especially whether or not older people experience dependency.

The health and social services are key agencies in the social construction of dependency in old age. These services and the professionals and other staff working in them have a significant impact on the welfare of older people and, by the approaches they adopt to the assessment of need, the provision of treatment and the delivery of care, they can play a large part in determining whether older people are either dependent or interdependent adults, whether they are empowered or powerless. This sort of analysis, combined with other developments in the mature European welfare states, has begun to set a new agenda in the relationship between welfare professionals and older people and, therefore, also provides a challenge for professional education and training. This focuses on the prevention or deconstruction of dependency in old age. Indeed, one of the most important issues now confronting all advanced health and long-term care systems is how to promote the participation of older people and their family carers in the processes of treatment and care (a point I return to below).

Institutional ageism

The idea that old age is in some respects a social construction, defined by policy and practice, represents a direct challenge to the crude medical model of old age as a period of inevitable deterioration and irreversible decrescence. Nonetheless, it is the negative view of old age as a disease that has dominated health and social care provision for the last fifty years. Old age has been 'medicalised', and this has reinforced dependency-creating structures and attitudes, even though, ironically, the medical profession itself plays a small role in the lives of older people. This is not to suggest that the social exclusion of older people can be blamed on the medical profession or that all sub-specialities have the same view of old age. However, the medical or disease model has exerted a disproportionate influence on health and social services provision and has helped to generate, as well as legitimate, different forms of age discrimination. Thus it is the interaction of the medical model and ageism that has had negative consequences for older people. Five main ones may be highlighted.

First of all, old age has been regarded, negatively, as being synonymous with either disease or loss of function, and older people have been treated as a homogeneous group. Although there are associations between advanced old age and disability and ill-health, these relationships are neither automatic or linear (OPCS 1988). Thus, even among very elderly people, it is a minority who suffer from severe disability and ill-health. For example, just over half of people aged eighty-five and over are able to go out of doors and walk down the road on their own, two-thirds are able to manage stairs. Although some three-fifths of men aged over sixty-five and two-thirds of women report a long-standing illness, the incidence is concentrated in the older age groups and does not represent a significant limitation on activity for the majority. Older people experience a higher than average incidence and duration of acute illness, restricting activities of men over seventy-five for an average of forty-seven days per year compared with twenty-three days for men of all ages. The figures for women over seventy-five are forty-seven and twenty-nine days, respectively (OPCS 1995). On average, older people consult their GP twice as often as younger people. The prevalence of moderate or severe cognitive impairment rises steeply with advanced old age – from 2.3 per cent in those aged sixty-five to seventy-four, to 7.2 per cent in those aged seventy-five to eighty-four, and to 21.9 per cent for those aged eighty-five and older. Thus, even though the minority experiencing severe illness or functional loss can be a significant one – and, in view of the numbers involved, this has serious implications for the health and social services – it is nonetheless a minority even at advanced ages.

However, because of the influence of the disease model of ageing, there is a common tendency to regard disability and ill-health as a 'normal' feature of the ageing process. This can result in unnecessary restriction of activity and social exclusion if a condition is left untreated or is poorly diagnosed. Policy-makers have consistently downplayed and underestimated the impact of disability in old age, fearing the public expenditure consequences of providing compensation to this, the largest group of disabled people. As a result, older people are excluded from claiming certain social security benefits paid to younger disabled people, such as incapacity benefit and disability living allowance (Walker 1990a). Successive government ministers, including Ministers for the Disabled, have tried to pass off functional impairment as a 'normal' part of growing older (Henwood 1990), even though there is plenty of evidence that it is not and that treatment and therapies can assist independence and participation.

Second, linked to this homogenisation of old age as a form of disease has been the dominance of institutional approaches to both treatment and social care. Of course, this institutional bias has a much wider impact on all those suffering from chronic conditions but, with regard to older people, the emphasis in health services on acute and curative medicine has meant that the particular needs of this group for preventive and rehabilitative services have not been fully catered for. These latter services have traditionally occupied a low status within the NHS hierarchy and they have been underresourced. The consequence for older people is that they are experiencing unnecessary levels of restriction on their activities, either because insufficient attention has been paid to prevention or because new rehabilitation techniques, for example for stroke patients, are not made widely available. There will always be an imperative to ration health resources, but the point being made here is that an excessive focus on acute and curative medicine disadvantages and, indirectly, discriminates against older people, and this results in social exclusion.

Third, more direct forms of institutional age discrimination, or ageism, flow from the interaction between the disease model of old age and the underlying ageism of society as a whole. Within the health service there is a growing catalogue of examples of direct discrimination against older people. One such example is screening for osteoporosis (Henwood 1990). More than 46,000 people a year in England and Wales suffer hip fracture, and three-fifths of them are women aged seventy-five and over. Roughly one-quarter of them die as a result of their injuries and complications, and many more fail to regain full mobility. Despite the fact that the risk factors and prevalence of osteoporosis are well known, as are the severe consequences of fractures, screening and preventive therapies for this condition have a low priority. In effect, this is a form of discrimination against older people and older women in particular. Another example is screening for cervical cancer, which specifically excludes older women even though 40 per cent of deaths from cancer of the cervix in England occur in women aged sixty-five and over. In fact, discrimination against older people 'appears to be a general feature of cancer treatment' (Henwood 1990: 54). Roughly half of all new malignancies occur in people aged over sixty, yet medical research and treatment has neglected this age group. People over the age of seventy are excluded from most clinical trials of cancer treatment, and older people 'receive either untested treatments, inadequate treatments, or even none at all, at the whim of their clinician' (Fentiman 1990: 1020).

Turning from health to the social services, researchers have noted the different perceptions of social care workers towards the care of children and older people and, more importantly, that different standards were being set for these two groups. In particular, social workers place working with older people way below work with children. This age discriminatory service hierarchy was built into the UK welfare system when, early in the post-war period, it was decided that community living was preferable to institutional care for all groups. However, in the case of children, this principle was put into legislation, but it was not with regard to older people.

The concern to maintain and foster family life evident in the Children Act was completely lacking in the National Assistance Act. The latter made no attempt to provide any sort of substitute family life for old people who could no longer be supported by their own relatives. Institutional provision was accepted without question.

(Parker 1964: 106)

Domiciliary services for older people were not regarded as a priority and were left largely to the voluntary sector (Means and Smith 1994: 25).

Fourth, the exercise of professional power usually means the exclusion of older people and their family carers from discussions about their own care, thereby disempowering them. Often professional autonomy has been taken as meaning that decisions could be made without the direct involvement of those most affected by them. In other words, health and social care are usually regarded as being the province of experts. Thus, as a result of the continuing domination of the medical model of treatment, which focuses excessively on the professional/service user relationship, service providers frequently employ very limited conceptions of both care and family carers.

With regard to care, there is a persistent reliance, by professionals assessing need, on the physical functioning and dependency of the cared-for person as the main eligibility criterion for services, which inevitably leads to other sources of carer stress being ignored. Furthermore, service providers' models of care are inherently reductionist, focusing usually on the physical aspects of care (Nolan *et al.* 1996). Often assessment processes break down the caring relationships into discrete tasks, in order to create convenient service-oriented categories of potential support (for example, with assessments based on physical functioning using the Activities of Daily Living scale). This approach fragments the caring experience and prevents an holistic picture from emerging. Thus both assessment processes and the services subsequently provided often fail to account for the dynamic, contextual and longitudinal dimensions of family care (Qureshi and Walker 1989). The results are a failure to understand the caring relationship, the meaning of care to those providing it, and consequently, an underestimation of carers' needs.

Carers themselves do not look upon what they do in straightforward task-based terms. Often caring is 'invisible', in that it does not include overt behaviour and is not always apparent to the person being cared for. The reason is that many carers seek to preserve the dignity and self-esteem of the older person by downplaying their dependency and keeping from them details of all the things that have to be done on their behalf (Qureshi and Walker 1989; Nolan *et al.* 1996). Thus, when service providers ask older people about the care they receive from family members, they are likely to get an incomplete picture.

It is not surprising, therefore, that some professionals also hold very limited conceptions of family carers. In practice, there are four main approaches taken by home care and other providers towards carers (Twigg and Atkin 1994: 11–15). First of all they may be superseded, when services take over their functions. Second, they may be regarded as 'resources' by professionals where services make assumptions about the availability of family carers. There is a clear danger here that carers will be exploited by the service providers, who use their presence to justify not providing a service. Third, carers may be regarded as 'co-clients', which recognises their need but subordinates them to the service provider. Not surprisingly, carers are not happy with this approach. Fourth, they may be treated as 'co-workers'. This model carries with it a danger that alliances between paid workers and family carers may disempower the person being cared for.

The common tendency to exclude family carers is a function of the organisational model which is implicit within service delivery and training regimes within the health and social services. In practice we may distinguish two forms of service organisation at the opposite ends of a continuum: bureaucracy and empowerment (see Table 9.1). In operational terms, the bureaucratic model may be said to enhance exclusion and dependency, in both physical and political terms (Walker 1982), while the empowerment model emphasises the interdependent status of older people as requiring assistance but with the right to autonomous decision-making. If we educate and train those working with older people in a bureaucratic mode, that will be the way they act in their practice.

Table 9.1 Models of service organisation

Bureaucratic model	Empowerment model
service/provider orientated	user orientated
inflexible	responsive
provider-led	needs-led
power concentrated	power sharing
defensive	open to review
conservative	open to change
input orientated	outcome orientated

The empowerment or user-centred approach aims to involve older service users in the development, management and operation of services as well as in the assessment of need (Croft and Beresford 1990, Walker 1992). The intention is to provide users and potential users with a range of realisable opportunities to define their own needs and the sort of services they require to meet them. Both carers and cared for are regarded as potential service users. Ideally, services would be organised to respect users' rights to self-determination, normalisation and dignity. They would be distributed as a matter of right rather than discretion, with independent inspection and appeals procedures, and would be subject to democratic oversight and accountability.

This is not to suggest that all professionals and para-professionals operate from a bureaucratic perspective, but this is a strong tendency in formal health and social care services. However, some social care professionals are beginning to question traditional models of training which emphasise professional autonomy and are seeking ways of working that are less oppressive and more open to user involvement (Ward and Mullender 1991). (An important contribution to this self-questioning in the fields of both home care and residential care for older people was made by Norman 1980.)

This transition is at an early stage, but already there are examples of service providers attempting to develop user-centred methods that emphasise, at the very least, the right of service users to be consulted. Some practitioners and social services departments are attempting to create partnerships in social work practice and social care in which older people are seen as active co-producers (Fisher and Marsh 1993, Warren and Walker 1992). There are also more radical examples of attempts to empower service users, including older people, to make their own decisions about care (Barnes 1997), an issue that I will return to in the third main section.

Fifth, the medical or disease model of ageing has helped to legitimate a negative perception of older people at the macro-political level. The combination of this inherently negative approach, an age-discriminatory culture, and the ideologically driven desire of politicians to limit public expenditure has created an alarmist 'demography of despair' in some quarters concerning the costs of population ageing. In Europe this pessimistic politics has concentrated on the future cost of pensions and reached its most extreme form in the UK in the 1980s (Walker 1990b). In the USA it has spawned a debate about the respective rights of the young and old to health care and, specifically, about whether limits should be set on the health services made available to older people (Callahan 1987, Howse 1998). We have already seen that older people in the UK are systematically excluded from some medical procedures and treatments; however, there has hardly been any public debate on this issue.

Marketisation and exclusion

It is not possible to blame the neo-liberal inspired policies of the 1980s and early 1990s for the exclusion of older people from health services and their disempowerment as service users. There are underlying age discriminatory processes which stretch back to the formation of the NHS. However, the likelihood that older people will experience exclusion has increased over the last two decades.

For more than thirty years in the UK there was political consensus on the care of older people: the main policy goal was community care and the dominant provider, as well as funder, was the public sector. The consensus was broken in the 1980s when, among other things, the government encouraged a rapid growth in private residential and nursing homes (a trebling of private residential homes between 1984 and 1994 and an eight-fold increase in nursing homes, with a near halving of public homes) and introduced a quasi-market with a strong bias towards private provision.

It was the imposition of market principles, coupled with the hurried removal of long-term care functions from the NHS and the forceful application of the crudest form of least-cost efficiency, that had such a deep impact on older people and their family carers. A tighter and tighter rationing of community care budgets has been imposed, with the result that in many places, support is available only for those in greatest need. Frail older people who, in previous decades, would have expected to receive some assistance are now being denied any. Instead family, friends and neighbours are being expected to provide care that should be the responsibility of the statutory authorities. There is a perverse incentive for older people to enter residential homes which universally results in increased dependency – there was a 120 per cent increase in the numbers entering residential and nursing homes in just four years (1992–96) – and the restrictions on fee levels, coupled with the enforcement of the more stringent means-test, has forced relatives and older people themselves to contribute towards the cost of long-term care. There are numerous instances of older people selling their homes to finance residential care, and it is estimated that 40,000–50,000 per annum will be forced to do so. This major policy development was never discussed openly, it never figured in an election campaign, yet it has enormous implications for intergenerational relationships within the family. Private residential home owners have legitimate causes for complaint as their fee levels are capped, and the levels of dependency of those they are caring for increase, but they are not being transferred to nursing homes.

Despite the huge amount of rhetoric about the new role of the health and social services consumer and listening to the views of carers, the fact is that the vast majority of older people, particularly those being discharged from hospital, do not have any choice in the matter of their care. Local authority care managers have been put in an impossible position of being expected to take on board the views of users while having to keep within budgets that are declining relative to the growth in need created by population ageing. What was trumpeted in the debate around the NHS and Community Care Act (1990) as a new needs-led service has quickly reverted to one which attempts to meet needs within tightly controlled and inadequate budgets. Not surprisingly, resources are being focused only on those with the most pressing needs and, as a consequence, the possibility of preventive and rehabilitative work is being closed off.

The marketisation of health and social care and other related government policies have added five new problems to the long-standing deficiencies of community care in the UK. First, there is a disincentive for the NHS to provide intensive long-term support. The central guidance is clear: only people with 'complex or multiple health care needs...requiring...specialist or nursing supervision' fall within the NHS remit. Intensive long-term support following acute treatment is defined as social care. However, resources have not been shunted with patients and costs. Despite the rhetoric about transferring resources from hospitals to community, the historical distribution remains remarkably resilient, and power within the NHS continues to reside in institutions. In some areas community health staff have been reduced.

Second, there are strong incentives for local authorities to ration the amount of care they provide, for example by disputing responsibility with the NHS; by purchasing residential care, whether or not it is appropriate, if cost recovery is more likely than from domiciliary care; racheting down the quality of care to minimise costs (the fate of Neighbourhood Support Units in Sheffield, see Walker and Warren 1996); targeting resources only on people with the highest levels of disability, at the expense of those with lower levels of needs, and thereby excluding the possibility of a preventive role for social care; capping the costs of care; and targeting provision on those without relatives providing care, thereby neglecting the importance of supporting family carers and recognising their needs. All of these rationing devices have serious consequences for equity of treatment between different older people and carers.

It is clear that resources are being targeted more and more narrowly. Terms such as 'high risk' and 'high need' are becoming familiar in local authority guidelines (and there are ready-made social science tools to enable such distinctions to be made). Official figures show that, in 1996, there was a drop of 5 per cent in the number of people receiving domiciliary care and a fall of 11 per cent in day care. In other words, the care gap is growing. According to the *General Household Survey 1995* (OPCS 1997), more than half of older people living alone are getting no help with the domestic tasks they cannot perform. This is despite a substantial increase in the role of the private sector in domiciliary care – from 2 per cent in 1992 to 29 per cent in 1995. It seems that the existing casualty role of social care has been further residualised and has become the very last resort.

Third, there has been a massive and rather panicky increase in charges for community care services and substantial variations in charging between local authorities. Of course charging is not new, what is new is the range of services local authorities are charging for and the high levels of the charges. A recent study has shown that the main pressure for increased charging has come from the funding shortfall, and there has been very little consultation and very little information for service users (Chetwynd *et al.* 1996). Some means testing systems are so complex that they have baffled front line providers as well as users. It is well known that older people are particularly likely to be discouraged by means tests.

Fourth, there are variations between authorities as to where the boundary is being drawn between the responsibilities of the NHS and SSDs. There are no national standards. Therefore, two older people in identical circumstances may find themselves being treated differently because they live in different areas. There is something of a lottery about the service response users and carers may get.

Fifth, there are financial incentives towards the provision of large-scale residential units (the return of the warehouse). A recent study found that the average cost of intensive home care is £157 per week (£140 after charges) compared with a net cost of residential care of £133 (after reducing the gross cost by at least £96.50 to account for the social security residential allowance and the residents' state pension). Furthermore, it is not possible to place a charge against an older person's property asset in respect of domiciliary services but authorities can do so in respect of residential care costs. In other words, there is still a perverse incentive favouring residential care. The cost incentives favour warehousing too. A 1995 survey by the British Federation of Care Home Proprietors found that 65 per cent said they would go out of business if local authorities imposed a requirement for single rather than shared rooms. Only 10 per cent of them supported single occupancy for all residents. In fact, an ADSS survey in 1995 found that only 6 per cent of authorities impose a blanket requirement for single rooms and 44 per cent required 80 per cent of rooms to be single. A 1995 survey by Counsel and Care found that 95 per cent of older people who live in their own homes said they would want a single room if they entered residential care.

The imposition of market principles in health and social care provision and the tighter and tighter rationing of resources under the Thatcher and Major governments have exacerbated the exclusion of older people and their family carers. Ironically, these policies have been promoted by rhetoric concerning increased choice for social care 'consumers'. In reality, this has meant the promotion of the private sector of care with public subsidies and the residualisation of the state as a direct provider (Walker 1989). But the previous government's policy did emphasise flexibility, plurality and choice.

In the White Paper *Caring for People*, 'choice' was defined as giving people a greater individual say in how they live their lives and the services they need to help them' (DOH 1989: 4). This was to be achieved in two main ways: a comprehensive process of assessment and care (or case) management, which 'where possible should induce [the] active participation of the individual and his or her carer', and a more diverse range of non-statutory providers, among the benefits of which is held to be a 'wider range of choice of services for the consumer' (ibid.: 10, 22). Unfortunately, however, these laudable aims existed largely in rhetoric rather than practice. The two main reasons for this are, on the one hand, that the policy derived from an ideology which is averse to making the increases in public expenditure necessary to realise the stated goals of participation and choice; and, on the other, that the model of participation on which the policy was based is a very shallow form of consumerism (Walker 1992, Barnes and Walker 1996).

This consumer model underlying the previous government's strategy derives from a limited form of supermarket-style consumerism which assumes that, if there is choice, service users will automatically have the power of 'exit', that is, the power to give up consuming a particular product (Hirschman 1970). Of course, even if this is true in markets for consumer goods, in the field of health and social care many older people are frail and vulnerable; they are not in a position to 'shop around' and have no realistic prospect of exit. Moreover, research suggests that the association between marketisation and choice is often false (Bradshaw and Gibbs 1988). Private markets create choice only for those that can afford the full range of goods or services on offer, and private forms of care are no less dominated by bureaucratic rules and professional assessments than their public counterparts. Also quasi-markets are difficult to operationalise in the context of a monopoly purchaser and without the wasteful purposive duplication of service suppliers (Hoyes and Means 1991).

Underlying this consumerist model of social care are two questionable assumptions. First, it is assumed that monopolies can only operate in the public sector. However, as far as – for example – an isolated and frail older recipient of home or residential care, either public or private is concerned, her provider may well be the monopoly power because she has no realistic alternative. Having a range of theoretical alternatives will not make the consumer sovereign if she cannot exercise effective choice. Second, it is assumed that direct payment opens the door to participation by conferring power. But a financial transaction does not necessarily mean the bestowal on the purchaser of either influence or control over the provider. By definition, the relationship between the social care provider and the user is an unequal power relationship and, regardless of whether or not there is an exchange of money, it is the provider that holds the power.

The consumerist perspective derives from a crude and narrow economic rationale and, not surprisingly, the organisational forms arising from it are managerial, displaying, for example, overriding concern with cost efficiency and cost containment. This managerialism inevitably reinforces the power of professionals, for instance through forms of case management which see older users as passive receivers of care – 'clients' to be 'managed'. In fact the only way that frail and vulnerable service users can be assured of influence and power over service provision is if they themselves are guaranteed a 'voice' in the organisation and management of services. This would, in turn, ensure that services actually reflected their needs. Because of its restricted economistic underpinnings the consumer perspective also perpetuates very limited constructions of both the needs of older people and the potential of social care. The needs of older people are viewed negatively in terms of dependency, and the role of social care is confined to that of maintenance or tending rather than prevention or rehabilitation.

Barriers to the inclusion and empowerment of older people

How can the health and social care services respond to the challenges of involving older users in the production of their own welfare and empowering them? It must be acknowledged that there are formidable institutional barriers to the inclusion and empowerment of older people and other service users.

First, there are organisational principles and structures that can exclude service users. For example professionalisation and, in particular, a still dominant model of training that encourages professionals and para-professionals to regard themselves as experts operating autonomously. Then there are power differentials, based on knowledge, control over resources, social class and other factors, between health and social services workers and powerless older users and potential users.

Second, there is resistance to change based partly on self-interest, partly on uncertainty, partly on lack of skill, and partly on insufficient resources to enable staff to invest the time necessary to learn new approaches and implement them. User participation has been described as 'putting the pain back into the system' (Jowell 1990), and no individual or system subjects itself to pain willingly. Past failures may increase an agency's reluctance to contemplate change. Research among service providers and service users aged seventy-five and over found that the main worry among home care workers about developing more open and participative ways of working was the fear that demand would be created that could not be fulfilled. This is a reasonable concern, but one that could be shared openly with users. Home carers also felt that they lacked the specialist skills to deal with complex relationships between informal carers and cared-for. Home Help Organisers were hard pressed managing 2–300 home carers and said they lacked the time and space to think and work flexibly (Allen *et al.* 1992).

Third, there are often major practical and personal barriers to participation facing older users themselves, for example poverty and low incomes. The poverty rate among older people in the UK is higher than in other comparable northern EU countries (Walker *et al.*

1993). There may be physical or mental obstacles to participation and communication, such as dementia, meaning that older service users may require significant assistance and support to enable them to become involved. Racial and other forms of discrimination may deter some groups of potential service users.

Facing the challenges of older people's right to participation

What steps are necessary if health and social care services are to overcome these barriers to user participation and move towards the inclusion and empowerment of older people and, thereby, the deconstruction of dependency in old age?

In the first place it is necessary to recognise that, while the private and voluntary sectors may extend choice in social care, they cannot fully substitute for the public sector. Only the public sector can guarantee legal rights to services. Thus, if the market and the voluntary sector provide exit for service users, at least in theory, then the democratic machinery of the state is the only provider that can ensure users have the right to a voice (Hirschman 1970). Regardless of how large the independent sector becomes, the state must always play an important role in regulation, protecting the rights of frail and vulnerable older people and guaranteeing access to services.

Second, change is necessary in the organisation and operation of formal services. The concept of social support networks is particularly helpful in emphasising the need for formal and informal helpers to cooperate, share tasks and decision-making and 'interweave' with each other (Whittaker and Garbarino 1983). This means, for example, that care would take the form of coordinated 'packages' in which a social care worker would act as part of a team, often as the key worker. It implies, too, that teamwork consists of professionals, para-professionals, service users and informal carers.

In addition, health and social care providers need to develop explicit strategies for the inclusion of older people. The essential ingredients of such a strategy are positive action – to provide users and potential users with support, skills training, advocacy and resources – so that they can make informed choices; and access – the structures of the agency must afford opportunities for genuine involvement (Croft and Beresford 1990: 24).

Third, there should be an open policy of supporting family carers and regarding their needs as having the same priority as those of older people (recognising, of course, the frequent conflicts of interest involved). In other words, carers also have a right to participation. The most important method of supporting carers is the level and quality of the services provided to their older relative (Twigg *et al.* 1990). Thus if it is possible to maximise the well-being and independence of the older service user, this will relieve both the physical strain and the mental anxiety of the informal carer. This emphasises the important, yet often neglected, roles of social care in the prevention of dependency and traumas such as carer breakdown, and in rehabilitation. Thus social care itself can make a positive contribution to the participation potential of both older people and their informal helpers (Levin *et al.* 1983).

Fourth, change must be initiated in professional values and attitudes within the formal sector, so that cooperation and partnership with users is regarded as a normal activity. This does not mean that service provision must be deprofessionalised if user participation is to flourish. But rather that the attitudes and roles of professionals and para-professionals must change in order to share power with users.

Fifth, the previous two points suggest a major transformation in training and retraining for health and social care personnel. Thus the emphasis in training would shift away from autonomous expertise and individual diagnosis towards skills for working in partnership with users and encouraging community participation. The research by Allen and her colleagues (1992), referred to earlier, shows that home carers lacked the skills to operate in a more flexible, open and empowering way. Other UK research, on partnership approaches in social work, found that social workers were reluctant to give up control over problem definition which they regarded as de-skilling. They found it hard to shift their conception of professional expertise towards problem negotiation (Fisher and Marsh 1993).

Sixth, user participation is not a cheap option, it is usually time-consuming and costly. Therefore there is a need for increased resources in social care, not only to improve the choice and quality of services but also to ensure that they provide sufficient space for user involvement. In Allen *et al.*'s research on service provision to people aged seventy-five and over, many Home Help Organisers were 'struggling' with the move from a service-led to a needs-led culture. They wanted to offer a person-centred approach to the delivery of care, but this seemed to slip from their grasp as they recognised the overwhelming economic and political pressure to ration and prioritise services (Allen *et al.* 1992).

Thus the key components of an effective policy of user participation are: resources, training, information, equal access, clear rights and entitlements, forms of redress, time and, if necessary, advocacy (Croft and Beresford 1990: 42). In addition, if local initiatives are to contribute to wider policy development then there must be research and evaluation and the dissemination of good practice.

'Empowerment' is an abstract term that must be turned into reality by a programme of practical action and innovation. This means commitment at all levels and the allocation of sufficient resources to put it into practice. It means recognising cultural diversity and, therefore, constructing different approaches for different local settings. The assessment process is crucial: do older people and their carers have a full opportunity to articulate their own needs in their own terms – not in service provider's predetermined categories? Are they made to feel inferior to service providers/ assessors or equal to them? If people cannot articulate their own needs, are there advocates to help them? Do staff act like 'experts' or in a way that suggests that they have something to learn from the real experts? Is there scope for self or group assessment?

As a guideline for those health and social care workers who are contemplating changing their practice in order to try more empowering approaches, particularly with frail older people, Barnes and Walker (1996) have elaborated eight key principles for such action:

1   *Empowerment should enable personal development as well as increasing influence over services,* i.e. the process should not be introduced only to benefit the professional group or service providers (in a 'top-down' way). An empowering approach should produce change in people as a result of the process of participation by, for example, reducing isolation and increasing confidence.

2   *Empowerment should aim to increase people's abilities to take control of their lives as a whole, not just increase their influence over services,* i.e. the benefit of participation can extend beyond the service context. The experience of having one's ideas and opinions valued can encourage people to participate in other areas.

3   *Empowerment of one person should not result in the exploitation of others: either family members or paid carers,* i.e. there is the danger of increasing the burdens on family members. This emphasises the importance of professionals examining how they interact with family carers: as resources, as co-workers, as clients or as experts?

4 *Empowerment should not be viewed as a zero sum: a partnership model should provide benefits to both parties*, i.e. it is not simply a matter of shifting the balance of power between professionals and older people. There is potential for growth on both sides of the relationship – personal development and professional development (in the form of new skills and new ways of working).

5 *Empowerment must be reinforced at all levels within service systems*, i.e. the danger here is that users are kept to the periphery of services. If people are not given a voice in the allocation of services, they will become very cynical about consultation.

6 *Empowerment of those who use services does not remove the responsibilities of those who produce them*, i.e. it is *not* a matter of professionals handing over their responsibility for decision-making. People seek help from the health and social services because they want to benefit from the knowledge and expertise which professional training should confer.

7 *Empowerment is not an alternative to adequate resourcing of services*, i.e. sometimes authorities have engaged service users in consultation but have not allocated sufficient resources for service provision. This is exploiting the goodwill of users.

8 *Empowerment should be a collective as well as an individual process; without this people will become increasingly assertive in competition with each other*, i.e. the importance of emphasising the collective basis of the welfare state so as to avoid conflict between different groups of service users (e.g. across generations) and to ensure the ongoing support of citizens in general.

The changes necessary to empower older service users and their carers entail nothing short of a cultural revolution within the health and social services: the replacement of provider-led models of health and social care by a partnership in which users' needs are uppermost. This would bring benefits to both parties: older users seem to prefer a more flexible and open approach to service provision (Qureshi *et al.* 1989), while care staff would find their job more rewarding and, together, they may put a case for greater resources.

Conclusion

It is feasible, in theory at least, to envisage forms of health and social care provision in which older service users and their carers are involved at every level of service planning and delivery. However, there is substantial institutional inertia standing in the way of this inclusion and empowerment. This inertia can only be overcome by a refocusing of health and social care services away from acute medicine and casualty-style social care interventions towards a greater emphasis on public health, prevention and rehabilitation. This 'cultural revolution' would include a programme of action designed both to convince health and social care workers that a core component of their practice is the inclusion of older people and their family carers in all decisions concerning their care, and to provide them with the skills and resources to do so. An important part of this process would be age discrimination awareness training. The starting point is for policy-makers themselves to give priority to tackling the exclusion of older people and the ageism that underpins it.

References

Allen, I., Hogg, D. and Peace, S. (1992) *Elderly People: Choice, Participation and Satisfaction*, London: PSI.

Barnes, M. (1997) *Care, Communities and Citizens*, London: Longman.

Barnes, M. and Walker, A. (1996) 'Consumerism versus empowerment – a principled approach to the involvement of older service users', *Policy and Politics* 24, 4: 375–93.

Bradshaw, J. and Gibbs, I. (1988) *Public Support for Residential Care*, Aldershot: Avebury.

Callahan, D. (1987) *Setting Limits: Medical Goals in an Aging Society*, New York: Simon and Schuster.

Chetwynd, M., Ritchie, J., Reith, L. and Howard, M. (1996) *The Cost of Care*, York: JRF.

Croft, S. and Beresford, P. (1990) *From Paternalism to Participation*, London: Open Services Project.

Department of Health (DOH) (1989) *Caring for People*, London: HMSO.

Estes, C.L. (1979) *The Ageing Enterprise*, San Francisco: Jossey-Bass.

Fentiman, I.S. (1990) 'Cancer in the elderly: why so badly treated?', *The Lancet* April 28: 1020–2.

Fisher, M. and Marsh, P. (1993) *Readiness to Practice*, York: Joseph Rowntree Foundation.

Freidson, E. (1970a) *Professional Dominance*, New York: Atherton.

——(1970b) *Profession of Medicine*, New York: Dodd, Mead & Co.

Guillemard, A.M. (1980) *La Vieillesse et l'état*, Paris: PUF.

Henwood, M. (1990) 'No sense of urgency', in E. McEwan (ed.) *Age: The Unrecognised Discrimination*, London: ACE Books.

Hirschman, A. (1970) *Exit, Voice and Loyalty*, Cambridge, Mass.: Harvard University Press.

Howse, K. (1998) 'Health care rationing, non-treatment and euthanasia: ethical dilemmas', in M. Bernard and J. Phillips (eds) *The Social Policy of Old Age*, London: CPA.

Hoyes, L. and Means, R. (1991) *Implementing the White Paper on Community Care*, Bristol: SAUS.

Jowell, T. (1990) 'Care in the Community: making it happen', presentation to the DOH Conference.

Levin, E., Sinclair, I. and Gorbach, P. (1983) *The Supporters of Confused Elderly Persons at Home*, London: NISW.

Means, R. and Smith, R. (1994) *Community Care*, London: Macmillan.

Nolan, M., Grant, G. and Keady, J. (1996) *Understanding Family Care*, Buckingham: Open University Press.

Norman, A. (1980) *Rights and Risk*, London: Centre for Policy Studies on Ageing.

OPCS (1988) *The Prevalence of Disability Among Adults*, London: HMSO.

——(1995) *The General Household Survey 1994*, London: HMSO.

——(1997) *The General Household Survey 1995*, London: HMSO.

Parker, J. (1964) *Local Health and Welfare Services*, London: Allen & Unwin.

Phillipson, C. (1982) *Capitalism and the Construction of Old Age*, London: Macmillan.

Qureshi, H. and Walker, A. (1989) *The Caring Relationship*, Houndmills: Macmillan.

Qureshi, H., Challis, D. and Davies, B. (1989) *Helpers in Case-Managed Community Care*, Aldershot: Gower.

Townsend, P. (1981) 'The structured dependency of the elderly: the creation of social policy in the twentieth century', *Ageing and Society* 1, 1: 5–28.

Twigg, J. and Atkin, K. (1994) *Carers Perceived: Policy and Practice in Informal Care*, Buckingham: Open University Press.

Twigg, J., Atkin, K. and Perring, C. (1990) *Carers and Services: A Review of Research*, London: HMSO.

Walker, A. (1980) 'The social creation of poverty and dependency in old age', *Journal of Social Policy* 9, 1: 49–75.

——(1982) 'Dependency and old age', *Social Policy and Administration* 16, 2: 115–35.

——(1989) 'Community care' in M. McCarthy (ed.) *The New Politics of Welfare*, London: Macmillan.

——(1990a) 'The benefits of old age?', in E. McEwan (ed.) *Age: The Unrecognised Discrimination*, London: ACE Books.

——(1990b) 'The economic "burden" of ageing and the prospect of intergenerational conflict', *Ageing and Society* 10, 4: 377–96.

——(1992) 'Towards greater user involvement in the social services', in T. Arie (ed.) *Recent Advances in Psychogeriatrics* 2, London: Churchill Livingstone.

Walker, A. and Warren, L. (1996) *Changing Services for Older People*, Buckingham: Open University Press.

Walker, A., Alber, J. and Guillemard, A-M. (1993) *Older People in Europe: Social and Economic Policies*, Brussels: Commission of the EC.

Ward, D. and Mullender, A. (1991) 'Empowerment and oppression: an indissoluble pairing for contemporary social work', *Critical Social Policy* 32, 21–30.

Warren, L. and Walker, A. (1992) 'Neighbourhood support units: a new approach to the social care of older people', in C. Victor and F. Laczko (eds) *Social Policy and Older People*, Aldershot: Gower.

Whittaker, J. and Garbarino, J. (eds) (1983) *Social Support Networks*, New York: Aldine.

Wilding, P. (1982) *Professional Power and Social Welfare*, London: Routledge.

10 Informational health networks

Health care organisation in the information age

Brian D. Loader

Introduction

The dramatic and fundamental economic and social changes that have occurred in all advanced capitalist societies in the final decades of the millennium have placed considerable pressures upon the role of the democratic welfare state as a means to deliver health care (Hurst 1992, Moran 1997). The seemingly insatiable demands being made upon publicly financed health care organisations have induced many governments to begin to question their responsibility for the direct provision of health services and to seek alternative organisational strategies for the delivery of health outcomes for their populations. In the academic world debate has crystallised around the contention that traditional bureaucratic organisations are insufficiently responsive to the requirements of the emerging global informational economies and are likely to be replaced by more flexible decentralised networks, whose primary means of operation is the processing of information, whose need for perpetual innovation in the achievement of its goals ensures the self-referential amendment of those means, and whose development is increasingly predicated upon new information and communications technologies (ICTs) (Hoggett 1990, 1991, Fox 1993, Castells 1996, 1997, 1998).

In the UK health domain, which will form the focus of this chapter, we have witnessed the most significant changes since the National Health Service (NHS) was established in 1948. These began with the introduction of the internal market (DOH 1989), followed by the advent of the New Public Health movement (DOH 1992, Petersen and Lupton 1996), and, more recently the New Labour administration's proposals set out in *The New NHS* (DOH 1997) and *Our Healthier Nation* (DOH 1998). Such developments can in part be understood as policy responses to the socio-economic restructuring of late capitalist societies. What all these policy initiatives share is a possible emerging consensus about the increasing transfer of responsibility for health from the state to the citizen. As such, they may be interpreted as a gradual, profound, but unsystematic trend towards a new form of health care organisation based upon a reformulation of the socio-economic relations between state, community and the citizen.

This chapter explores the contention that health care organisation is likely to manifest itself in the emergence of new organisational control paradigms (Hoggett 1994), moving from vertically integrated command and control structures towards self-regulation and decentralised autonomous control strategies. In particular, it is hypothesised that we may witness entirely new configurations of health care systems arising from home- and community-centred consumption, personal responsibility arising from self-risk analysis, and local networks of social support comprising a mixture of primary health care professionals, voluntary and community groups, and other statutory agents. I propose to call these new forms of health care organisation 'informational health networks' (IHNs).

The driving forces facilitating such a transformation are likely to be the continuing economic pressure upon politicians to contain public expenditure in the face of increasing demands being made upon health resources; the phenomenal and rapid developments in ICTs, in particular the synthesis of a range of information technologies such as telecommunications, computers, virtual reality, satellite, smart cards and other forms of informatics; and the growing pressure for change from social movements in a society increasingly characterised by greater social difference and diversity.

The effects of these combined factors, whilst impossible to predict with accuracy, may nonetheless be speculatively discerned in some of the current early consequences of organisational restructuring. It is possible to detect in the most recent reforms and accompanying policy debates a move away from the rationalist, paternalistic, centralist model of medical provision towards a more pluralistic system emanating from the community. A particular concern arising from this possible trend towards informational health networks is what the consequences may be for those who at present do not appear to be well placed to connect to the Net. The suggestion made here is that, at least in the short term, it is likely to reinforce existing health inequalities and exclude large segments of the population who are unable actively to promote their own health.

'There's an east wind coming...'

Health policy is not produced from some kind of socio-economic *tabula rasa*. As Rudolph Klein persuasively reminds us, the origins of the NHS itself are to be found in a broad political consensus about post-war health policy objectives:

> Nothing is more remarkable than the shared assumption that the health service should be both free and comprehensive – and that it should be based upon the principle of the collective provision of services and the pooling of financial risks through the public financing of the service.
>
> (Klein 1995: 24)

Klein also emphasises the point that, whilst there may have been consensus between competing interests about the policy 'ends', this did not preclude an energetic and intense debate about the 'means' to be adopted for achieving the desired objective (ibid.: 25). For perhaps a little over three decades the consensus for a largely nationally financed and delivered health care system that was comprehensive, universal and free at the point of delivery remained practically unchallenged. Certainly there were debates about the cost of the NHS and periodic reforms of its organisation, but these never undermined the socially inclusive ideal of the health service.[1] By the final decades of the twentieth century, however, a colder socio-economic environment was beginning to emerge which would test the fabric of Britain's collectivist NHS.

Three environmental changes can be identified which are of particular significance to health care organisation: the trend towards a global competitive economy and the corresponding development of new organisational forms; the emergence of new ICTs; and the development of new social structures.

Economic restructuring and new organisational forms

In his major work on the Information Age, Manuel Castells (1996, 1997, 1998) portrays the economic restructuring of capitalist societies as being distinguished by the development of an 'informational economy' and the process of 'globalisation'. The new economy:

> is informational because the productivity and competitiveness of units or agents in this economy (be it firms, regions, or nations)

fundamentally depend upon their capacity to generate, process, and apply efficiently knowledge-based information. It is global because the core activities of production, consumption, and circulation, as well as their components (capital, labour, raw materials, management, information, technology, markets) are organised on a global scale, either directly or through a network of linkages between economic agents.

(Castells 1996: 66)

This advent of a global informational economy is considered to have significant implications for the role and sustainability of the Keynesian welfare state (KWS). First, 'there is a clear disjuncture between the formal authority of the state and the spatial reach of contemporary systems of production, distribution and exchange which often function to limit the competence and effectiveness of national political authorities' (Held 1995: 127). The remarkable developments of new ICTs appear to erode the boundaries of national economies and thereby lay them open to increased competition from multinational companies, which focus their operations at the global and regional rather than national level. Thus Britain's relative industrial decline has made recent successive governments increasingly concerned, both about their limited capacity to control financial markets, raise tax revenue, attract investment, provide industrial support, and about the level of public expenditure directed towards welfare. Simultaneously, the pressure for increased spending on health care has been pushed by the costs of a labour-intensive (despite a large percentage of low-paid employees) sector, the rising numbers of older people in the population, and the inflationary price of medical technology, all of which are likely to remain a central concern for government.

Second, as the whole basis of Keynesian demand management is called into question by this process of globalisation, so the future role of the state in the informational economy becomes foregrounded. In particular, the rigidity and costs of collectivist welfare provision come to be seen as a barrier to economic recovery rather than as a basis for economic growth, through the provision of a healthy educated workforce; social cohesion based upon redistributive taxation, social security and universal services; and economic demand through increased public expenditure programmes. The search for alternative government economic policies has in part been guided by the response from corporate capitalism to the informational economy – principally, the creation of new organisational forms and processes and the concomitant rise of the flexible information worker. Rather than the pursuit of full employment and social cohesion through redistributive welfare rights, the state's role becomes reoriented to supporting international competitiveness by encouraging a flexible workforce, product innovation, continuous skilling, and personal responsibility (Jessop 1994).

New organisational forms

It has become a commonplace to suggest that we are witnessing the emergence of new organisational forms which are a consequence of the increased pace of change associated with the informational economy (Heydebrand 1989, Clegg 1990, Harrison 1994, Castells 1996). The vertically integrated corporate organisations that were suited to the more stable environments of the post-war world are gradually being replaced, it is contended, by the new flexible and flatter organisational forms, which are characteristic of the information age. 'It is,' remarks Castells, 'the convergence and interaction between a new technological paradigm and a new organizational logic that constitutes the historical foundation of the informational economy' (1996: 152).

What, then, are the main features of these new organisational forms? Typically, six characteristics may be emphasised as the emergent properties of the post-bureaucratic organisation.

1   Hierarchical structures become flattened and replaced by horizontal decentralised core–periphery networks of self-directed units. Castells describes the most advanced of these as 'network enterprises', whereby the boundaries of organisations become blurred and indeterminate through their interaction with other networks. Thus, he contends, 'the unit [of economic organisation] is the network, made up of a variety of subjects and organizations, relentlessly modified as networks adapt to supportive environments and market structures' (1996: 198).

2   This, in turn, has entailed a movement away from rigid, centralised, vertical control strategies towards flexible *remote control* practices characterised by devolving resources to decentralised units whilst simultaneously making them responsible for their own performance set against other competing units and/or centrally determined targets (Cooper 1992, Hoggett 1994).

3   These processes, whilst not originally instigated by the development of new technologies, have nonetheless become increasingly

enhanced by the capacity of ICTs to foster flexibility and coordination.

4   The increased competition as a result of the global informational economy has precipitated the shift away from mass production of standardised goods and services towards niche markets based upon organisational learning and continuous innovation.

5   A combination of the above factors requires the de-differentiation of the work process and the introduction of multi-skilled or polyvalent forms of work organisation. A particular premium is placed upon positions requiring the imaginative, creative, information and knowledge-based skills of the 'symbolic analysts' (Reich 1992).

6   The pressures for a responsive organisational form based upon the networked coordination of specialised self-directed units leads to the development of more democratic and participative management predicated upon high-trust relationships (Fox 1974, Fukuyama 1996).

For such authors as Clegg (1990) and Castells (1996), these features do not amount to a universal model of organisational conformation so much as 'a common matrix' (ibid.: 151) from which a rich variety of configurations may develop according to such factors as location, culture, social structure or technological development. What they represent, however, is the potential emergence of a new template that challenges and gradually replaces the 'bureaucratic' as the dominant form of organisation.

Fierce debates and controversies have, however, surrounded these theoretical contentions suggesting the arrival of a new organisational paradigm. Whether in the guise of a Fordist/Post-Fordist, modernist/postmodernist duality, or in the more recent variants of the 'enterprise network', a number of important criticisms have been levelled at these propositions. Limited space precludes a detailed examination of all the complex arguments in this chapter, but it is nonetheless necessary to mention some of the suggested limitations.[2]

First, there is the accusation that these theories are constructed at a high level of abstraction and are consequently too general to be of any meaningful explanatory use. Second, they seem to be based upon a limited (although perhaps growing) number of empirical instances of high-profile companies such as Benetton and Toyota and may not stand up to more widespread examination. For example, the issue of flexibility has attracted a number of critical responses both to its assertion of a 'flexible labour force' and to the notion of the 'flexible firm'. Third, in some variants they have further been alleged to promote a form of technological determinism whereby the logic of capitalist development precludes any place for human choice or resistance. Lastly, the above concerns lead to a more cautionary stance about the degree to which new organisational structures and practices represent a sharp discontinuity with past processes. In particular some commentators have observed how the new control strategies focused on performance measurement may represent a continuity with the modernist scientific management theories of Frederick Taylor (Pollitt 1990).

Whilst recognising the contentious nature of these new models of organisation, and accepting that much more empirical work is still to be done before more conclusive modelling can be undertaken, it is equally important to be aware of their force as an emerging orthodoxy (see Webster and Robins 1998). In this context, a number of writers have alluded to attempts by policy-makers to draw lessons from private enterprise as a basis for reforming public sector institutions (Hoggett 1990, Stoker 1989, Murray 1991). As we will consider later, it is as an emergent template that it may be instructive, as a means of deciphering both the restructuring of health care organisation in Britain in recent years and some of its possible trajectories in the future. Thus, whatever the theoretical weaknesses of particular formulations, it is important that we do not underestimate the enormous overall influence that such perceived developments may have for policy formulation.

Information and communications technologies

Alongside the emergence of the global informational economy, a second phenomenon of profound import for environmental change has been the impact of new ICTs. For some commentators, the combined influence of a variety of technologies, including microelectronics, computers, multimedia, telecommunications and genetic engineering amount to nothing less than a technological revolution on a scale similar to, if not greater than, the first Industrial Revolution (Dizard 1989, Negroponte 1995, Castells 1996). Its force for change is derived from the convergence of these once separate technologies into a coherent system based upon information as its primary resource and which is pervasive throughout all aspects of socio-economic interaction. Since information 'is an integral part of all human activity, all processes of our individual and collective existence are directly shaped (although certainly not determined) by the new technological medium' (Castells 1996: 61).

Highly sophisticated computer networks, such as the Internet, which enables millions of people to communicate electronically around the world by means of a range of synthesised computer and telecommunications technologies, illustrate some of the transforming qualities of the new ICTs. In the first place, the configuration of the network is characterised by unimaginable complexity of interaction, which is in constant transmutation as a consequence of unpredictable growth and the continuous innovative applications of the technology. It is the creative resources of its users that are responsible for claims that the Internet cannot be controlled and the fears of others that this may be true.[3]

In literature, such writers as William Gibson have portrayed a world in which humans can 'jack into the net' and almost fuse with the technology to produce a combined intelligence (1984). More prosaically, however, a principal feature of the new technologies is the potential they offer to generate continuous learning and innovation through critical feedback loops informing and directing further development on the basis of knowledge and acquired intelligence. Castells again:

> what characterizes the current technological revolution is not the centrality of knowledge and information, but the application of such knowledge and information to knowledge generation and information processing/communication devices, in a cumulative feedback loop between innovation and the uses of innovation.
>
> (1996: 32)

The source of this seemingly infinite flexibility and potential for development is derived from the unbounded nature of the network, which is transnational and operational across all time zones. As a result, such technologies stand at the forefront of the means to deconstruct our conceptions of time and space (Harvey 1990). It is now possible to communicate at any time to anywhere provided that the agent or organisation is online.[4] This is complemented by another dimension to the morphology of the electronic network which is that it enables many-to-many interactive communication in contrast to the more limited uses of telephony or the one-to-many broadcast technologies associated with mass media.

It is not difficult to see how these rapid and impressive technological developments have increasingly come to be seen as the main driving force behind the present socio-economic restructuring of the environment. As stated earlier, in its characterisation as an emerging global informational economy it is predicated upon electronic networks that link world-wide locations of production, distribution, innovation and consumption and that are based upon the processing and communication of information/knowledge. Moreover, the flexible and decentralised network enterprises which are said to be appearing as a response are not only enabled by ICTs to adapt through autonomous reflexive learning but also typically employ a large percentage of highly skilled information workers. The financial markets perhaps represent the most advanced incarnation to date of these trends.

The changing social structure

A third facet of environmental development, and one which also finds resonance with the techno-economic transformations described above, is the concurrent restructuring of UK society. The British population which witnessed the establishment of the NHS in the late 1940s was essentially characterised by a patriarchal social class structure. Indeed, the welfare state has often been crudely portrayed as the outcome of a settlement of the social conflict between the organised working class and the interests of capital. The former countenanced the alienating conditions of many working practices in exchange for the ameliorating consequences of a welfare state devoted to supporting the individual from 'the cradle to the grave'.

The intervening fifty years, however, have seen a number of significant modifying factors, giving rise to the view that we now live in a very different society. Wider enjoyment of the benefits of capitalism through growing working-class ownership of cars, domestic entertainment media, and property, and the establishment of foreign package holidays together with the opportunities and services afforded by the welfare state, were the consequence of rising productivity, expanding industrial output and increasing real personal incomes during the 1950s and 1960s. At the time these phenomena led to the proclamation that we were seeing the '*embourgeoisement*' of the working class, who were said to be losing their identity – a view which received strong opposition from the classic studies of the 'affluent worker' by Goldthorpe and Lockwood (Goldthorpe *et al.* 1969).

The male, white, urban domination of the social class structure received a further challenge from the changes to employment patterns. Of particular impact were the increasing numbers of women entering the paid labour market, together with the immigration of New Commonwealth employees to help satisfy the UK's shortage of labour. Moreover, these developments were accompanied by a shift in the employment structure away from manual and towards non-manual service sector jobs. Such changes were also matched by geographical movements of people from the inner cities to a variety of orbital suburban owner-occupied estates, peripheral public housing, and New Town developments. The consequences of these resettlement policies upon traditional working-class communities have been regarded by some as loosening social class ties and identity.

These social trends have gathered pace since the late 1970s with the deindustrialisation of many old manufacturing areas, creating high levels of unemployment and the continuing decline of what were regarded traditionally as full-time male jobs. Where economic recovery has taken place, primarily in the south of the UK, the jobs created have tended to be part-time ones in the service sector taken mainly by women. As one might expect, such radical changes to employment opportunities, social geography and the increasing social, economic and political prominence of women, ethnic minorities and other social groups (hitherto largely omitted from earlier social analyses) have led to the proposition that social class alone is no longer an adequate classification of social differences.

The rich debate generated by such social transformations is beyond the scope of this short chapter. But two perspectives deserve further consideration for their importance as pointers to social action which may effect health service restructuring.

Consumerism and the commodification of welfare

One of the most influential propositions regarding change in the social relations of welfare is that there has been an increasing movement away from the collectivist state provision of publicly financed, universal services towards the 'recommodification' of welfare into individualised and privatised forms (Saunders 1984) – a gradual replacement of the 'welfare society' by the 'consumer society'. This is made possible, first, by the fragmentation of the working class by reorienting its classical relationship to the means of production and instead focusing its attention upon the consumption of state services. Ownership and control of the production system is replaced as the primary political objective by the desire to further the redistribution of society's resources through direct payment or provision by the state.

This consumption-centredness by the working classes is further reinforced by the increasing purchasing power experienced in the post-war years by affluent workers. For some commentators this has eroded social class solidarity based upon working conditions and led to a greater emphasis upon status as a basis for social differentiation (Marshall *et al.* 1985). Status is derived from consumption patterns and 'lifestyle' (Featherstone 1991). Thus:

> the critical forms of social experience for what previously has been understood to be the working class, while different from those of the service class in terms of quantity, are little different in terms of quality. If there are class boundaries at all they are based on exclusionary practices which seek to monopolise consumption advantages rather than acts of exploitation and appropriation in order to maintain control of production.
>
> (Crook *et al.* 1992: 121)

The advanced phase of this disaggregation of the class structure of society is the decline of state-provided welfare and the commodification of welfare to be obtained through the exercise of private transactions. This perspective has been notably portrayed by Peter Saunders, who observed that 'we are moving towards a dominant mode of consumption in which the majority will satisfy their requirements through market purchases (subsidised where necessary by the state) while the minority remain directly dependent on the state' (1984: 204).

Two separate but related consequences arise from the commodification of welfare services. In the first formulation, many consumers, unable to gain sufficient satisfaction from standardised, universal, bureaucratically organised state services, begin to distance themselves from collectively provided welfare and opt out of the system. Saunders maintains that increased home ownership and the sale of council housing provides evidence for what he believes will be a broader privatisation of other social services such as health and education (1984). Second, in perhaps a more pronounced version still, Bauman (1988) maintains that 'freedom' is increasingly expressed through consumerism in the market-place, in marked contrast to those whose activities are constrained and dependent upon the state. Both scenarios, however, depict the emergence of a significant social cleavage, with the majority of consumers satisfying their needs at the expense of a smaller excluded 'underclass', who are dependent upon public welfare.

The commodification of welfare thesis has been subject to objections. In the first place it has still to be established that individuals are in fact opting out of the welfare system. In the case of health services, whilst the private sector has indeed expanded over the past fifteen years or so, it remains a relatively minor proportion of UK health expenditure. More significantly, even those using private health facilities typically do so on a selective basis and thus do not 'leave the system'. A further criticism, voiced by Warde, is that the 'consumerist' model often 'bears an uncanny resemblance to contemporary orthodoxies of market research and invariably inflates the degree of recent change entailed' (1994: 228). What is lacking is the existence of reliable empirical evidence to support the claims for changing consumer behaviour patterns.

What can be discerned from this contested discourse is that the conception of individual private consumption as a higher good than publicly provided services will have a crucial bearing upon the way welfare is perceived, evaluated and restructured. This may be borne out by the curious paradox arising from the recent introduction of consumerism into the NHS, which had less to do with hearing the voice of the customer and was rather more the consequence of ministerial commands delivered through the managerial mouthpiece. As Klein remarks, 'the new rhetoric of consumerism is a response to top-down policies rather than to bottom-up demands' (1995: 238).

Social movements, difference and diversity

An alternative perspective, which relates the changes in UK society to developments in welfare restructuring, seeks to express these as complicated by the outcomes of social struggles and challenges of a range of social movements based around gender, race, and disability (Williams 1994). These social movements are not just organised around the distributional agenda of social class consumption but emerge in opposition to the organisation and professional power base of welfare institutions. As Fiona Williams asserts, 'both patriarchal and racialised processes have historically been challenged not necessarily by class struggle but by emancipatory movements of women and black and minority ethnic groups' (1994: 63). For many social groups, the welfare state settlement acted to institutionalise inequalities based upon male domination, nationalism, racism and homophobia (Williams 1989). Such an analysis is important for reminding us that, since its inception, the attempt by the NHS to provide universal provision has been on a conditional basis and that the nature of its practice has often acted to exclude many citizens.

Thus the restructuring of welfare cannot simply be regarded as a response to the weakening of social class solidarity but is also a consequence of the demands from other forms of social power. These came to express themselves in a number of counteracting activities, such as the establishment of well-women clinics, women's refuges and other types of voluntary provision, the development of equal opportunities policies within welfare organisations, and the radicalisation of some welfare professions themselves. The emphasis from this vantage point is that an understanding of welfare restructuring must include an acknowledgement of the impact of social struggle and resistance by diverse groups and different social movements. Its outcomes are 'a reflection of challenges and accommodations to a balance of power especially around class, race, and gender' (Williams 1994: 68).

Another value to this perspective is that it focuses attention upon the interplay of power relationships involved in the bargaining and competition for health policy outcomes. The domination of the medical profession within the NHS has been a recurrent theme over the years, with their power base emanating from the construction, ownership and restricted dissemination of medical knowledge. (McKeown 1976, Navarro 1986). As Fox contends, 'disciplines are both bodies of knowledge and strategies of power – meticulous methods by which docile bodies are manipulated and controlled' (1993: 62). The paternalistic nature of the doctor–patient relationship is grounded in an unequal discourse between the respective parties which cannot be militated by assertions of consumerism. The challenge to medical hegemony comes not from customer rights but rather from the empowerment derived from the construction of alternative competing discourses of health.

As with the previous interpretations considered above, this approach too may be inclined to overstate its impact upon changes in health policy. The power of the medical professions, whilst partially realigned between GPs and consultants, could not be said to have significantly diminished to date. Where power may be said to have shifted from professionals to managers, this could hardly be the main consequence of bottom-up pressure from social movements, any more than it is the product of consumerism.

The restructuring of the health service

The, albeit brief, consideration above of some of the enormous economic, technological and social changes currently underway is intended to provide a context for understanding the reformation of the NHS. In particular, I want to suggest that the competing and often partial interpretations of such profound restructuring provide the basis for policy formulations. This is not to suggest that the future organisation of health care is determined by these environmental changes, but rather that the debates around contested responses to them are informing deliberations about policy options.

A cursory appraisal of the 1991 NHS reorganisation (DOH 1989) could be regarded as an early response to wider socio-economic changes. The introduction of an internal market to divide the purchasing role from that of service providers represented a significant departure from the vertically integrated organisation of the health service. Henceforward, health authorities would be responsible for establishing contracts with a mixed market of health care providers and buying their services. This was an attempt to stimulate incentives to contain costs through increased efficiency, improve quality by establishing competition, and generating wider choice by enabling the use of alternative facilities. Through the adoption of a more businesslike culture,[5] the intention was to create an NHS which was more flexible and responsive to its environment.

Through their claim to be 'putting the patient first', the reforms also echoed the drive towards consumerism. As noted previously, however, this came not from the public but as a part of a top-down managerial strategy. In fact, the extent to which the customer has been empowered is somewhat limited to the freedom to change doctors and more recently the moderate guarantees outlined in the patients' charter. But the reforms did introduce another important dimension that was to improve the power bargaining status of GPs within this quasi-market (Le Grand 1990). Through the advent of budget-holding practices, many consultants have become increasingly accountable to GPs for the services they provide. This process has developed furthest where locality purchasing by a group of GPs has given them the potential to direct health services more closely to their patients' needs. As such, it could be taken to represent the beginning of a change in emphasis from domination by the hospital sector and towards community health.

It is not difficult, then, to regard such developments as examples of the breakdown of the bureaucratic model of health service delivery and its replacement by more decentralised, core–periphery forms of organisation. Together with the heightened use of devolved budgets, performance appraisal and clinical audit, it would further indicate the movement towards a strategy of remote control:

> Give managers and staff control over resources, make them accountable for balancing the books, add a framework of performance targets, and perhaps a few core values and mission statements, finally add a dash of competition and there you have it – a disaggregated, self-regulating form of public service production.
>
> (Hoggett 1994: 45)

Yet an appraisal of the 1991 reforms provides a mixed picture of continuity with the past, implementation failure, as well as genuine change. The transaction costs associated with the internal market and the concomitant rise in administration have both made it difficult to achieve the objective of containing costs or derive the benefits from contractual relationships. Choice for 'customers' has been restricted by location and the power-dependency relationship with their doctors. Rationing of services has continued on the basis of clinical decisions largely hidden from public view. The uneven spread of GP budget-holding has also led to assertions that the NHS's commitment to equity was being abandoned.

Towards an informational health network organisation?

However flawed, the 1991 reforms can be seen as a part of an ongoing process of experimentation and innovation, which takes as its framework the facilitating capacity of ICTs, the pluralism of the network structure, and the primary role of the citizen as having both obligations and rights. This interpretation is borne out in part by the pronouncements of the incoming Labour administration, as set out in *The New NHS* (DOH 1997), where any expectation that the new government would roll back the clock was dealt a firm blow. 'There will be no return to the old centralised command and control systems of the 1970s. That approach stifled innovation and put the needs of institutions ahead of the needs of patients' (ibid.: 10). Instead, the internal market is to be replaced by ' "integrated care" based on partnership and driven by performance' (ibid.: 5), cooperation is thereby substituted for competition, and the quasi-market is exchanged for a network system.

The new NHS also appears to continue the decentralising thrust towards locally directed services. Particular emphasis is placed upon the role of GPs and nurses as those best placed to understand patients' needs. This is reinforced by the desire to see more community 'advice and treatment in local surgeries and health centres with family doctors and community nurses working alongside other health and social care staff to provide a wide range of services on the spot' (ibid.: 6). Furthermore, it is recognised that these practices are facilitated by the introduction of the latest advances in medical informatics which, for example, enable more portable miniaturised equipment to assist in community-based diagnosis and treatment; online connectivity of GP surgeries and hospitals via NHSnet to support efficient communication of medical records, patient transfer, test results, access to current research and the like; and the use of telemedicine by which digital images can be passed across a network to link remote sites for the purposes of diagnosis or assistance with medical procedures.

The separation between the purchasing/commissioning and providing roles has also been retained. Fewer, larger Health Authorities will continue to be responsible for planning health services in partnership with local authorities, NHS Trusts and the intended Primary Care Groups (PCGs) by the construction of Health Improvement Programmes. They will also allocate and monitor funds to PCGs which will consist of all GPs and community nurses within an area. PCGs, building upon the experiments in locality purchasing, will control their own cash-limited budget, which they will be able to use for commissioning services from NHS Trusts or undertaking their own provision. NHS Trusts will be connected to the system by long-term service agreements with PCGs.

Of particular interest in *The New NHS* is the suggested decentralisation of responsibility for the management of individual health to the citizen. This appears in reference to home-based 'easier and faster advice and information for people about health, illness and the NHS so that they are better able to care for themselves and their families' (ibid.: 5). It manifests itself partially by the introduction of a twenty-four-hour telephone advice line supported by nurses, called NHS Direct. This is to be further supplemented in the future by providing access to information through the Internet and digital TV. Perhaps more predictably, the emphasis upon personal individual responsibility for health, though not the exclusive directive, is again restated in the government's Green Paper, *Our Healthier Nation* (DOH 1998).

Whilst still general in its ambitions and short on detail, *The New NHS* bears a striking resemblance to the characteristics of the new organisational forms outlined earlier. In this sense it can be considered as an early variant of an information health network (IHN), comprising a plurality of nodal points in the form of PCGs, Health Authorities, NHS Trusts, local authorities, and Regional and National Health Agencies. Increasingly, as the network adopts the informal voluntary and community sectors as service providers, social support agents as spaces for innovation and experimentation, the boundaries and roles separating health organisations become indeterminate. The informational network, following Castells (1996), becomes the unit of health care organisation.

But the proposals also indicate a possible future direction for health care organisation, which I have described elsewhere as 'welfare direct' – the replacement of 'rationally administered state provision, paternalistic professionally determined needs, and bureaucratic organisational delivery systems...[by] an emphasis upon fragmentation, diversity, and self reliance' (Loader 1998a: 220). Thus individual citizens, either acting alone or in groups, become incorporated into the network. A system of self-directed health care, with patients responsible for managing their own health care, emerges as they become a partner in their own informational health network.

Such a model of health care organisation does not necessarily require that the original objectives of the NHS for a comprehensive universal health service be discarded. It does, however, suggest that the relationship of the citizen to state will significantly alter, with individuals being required to take more responsibility for their health. For some this may be regarded as an inclusive strategy to enable patients to take more control of their own bodies and health (Pyper 1997). Indeed, the wealth of information, advice and social support increasingly available on the Internet provides a further connection to numerous other networks which could provide a means to challenge the dominant discourse and power base of the medical profession. Evidence-based research (as identified in *The New NHS*) can act to stimulate the negative information feedback loop required not only for the self-regulation of the health care units but also for the health risk analysis for individual lifestyle and activity.

What such an interpretation omits, however, is a consideration of power. Not all members of the network are equal in relation to each other. The agencies of the state, for example, still remain in a more powerful position *vis-à-vis* many of its citizens. The temptation to control public expenditure, for example, by transferring health care costs to the individual and/or community under the auspices of forcing people to be free from the dominance of the medical profession may prove irresistible. Similarly, some demands from the more articulate, information-rich sections of the population may lead to greater exclusion for those deprived of the requisite skills and access to the informational health network.

It could be countered that informational health networks are too general and flexible to have conceptual value. Certainly, it is unlikely that there will be any uniformity of such organisational forms, which will be configured according to different economic and social circumstances. Nevertheless, the primary features identified above are likely to inform health policy for at least the near future, which warrants that they should be taken seriously by students of health care organisation. In respect of social exclusion, they raise a number of pertinent questions for policy-makers and academics alike – in particular, those concerning the constellation of power relationships in the network. Are they, for example, gendered and racist? Who controls the flows of communication? Who facilitates the intensity of relations? How do they facilitate identity formulation? What are the consequences for the knowledge base of professionals?

Conclusion

I have attempted to suggest in this chapter that any meaningful understanding of recent policy reformulations of the UK's NHS should be regarded as responses to environmental socio-economic restructuring. Processes of globalisation and the advent of an informational economy have increasingly restricted the scope of government economic activity and challenged the post-war consensus about the role of the welfare state. It is likely that the continuing concern to impress the financial markets by controlling public expenditure will be matched by an emphasis upon shifting responsibility for social welfare from the state and towards the individual citizen. This will not negate social security for a targeted minority unable to meet their own needs through the employment market, familial support or private insurance provision. It does, however, represent a significant change to the welfare state orthodoxy of paternalistic rationalism to a perspective which champions independence and interdependence.

In the health policy arena, I have suggested that this emerging orthodoxy seems likely to manifest itself in a new organisational form which I have called an 'informational health network'. It represents the politics neither of the free market nor of the vertically integrated control and command structures of the traditional NHS model. Instead, it presents a site for contested perceptions of health care to be worked out. The relationship of the citizen to the NHS will remain an ambivalent one, mediated by power relations, opposition and resistance by competing social groups. The informational health network form of health care organisation both offers potential benefits to groups previously marginalised and raises the serious risk of reinforcing the current exclusion of those whose experience is constructed by their social circumstances.

Notes

1 This is not to suggest that all members of society were treated equally only that inclusiveness was a policy goal.
2 For a fairly comprehensive account of the Post-Fordist thesis as it applies to welfare, consider Burrows and Loader (1994). Good accounts of post-modern organisational theory can be found in Clegg (1990) and Reed (1992).
3 I have attempted to deal elsewhere with the hyperbole which frequently arises from discussions of the Internet. See Loader (1997).
4 I shall deal later with the issue of exclusion from the information network. See Loader (1998b).
5 Many of the new general managers and health authority chairs were recruited from the private sector. Moreover, the salary scales required to attract and retain those with the requisite skills very quickly rose in an attempt to mirror the private sector.

References

Bauman, Z. (1988) *Freedom*, Buckingham: Open University Press.
Burrows, R. and Loader, B. (eds) (1994) *Towards a Post-Fordist Welfare State?*, London: Routledge.
Castells, M. (1996) *The Information Age: Economy, Society and Culture*, Vol. I, *The Rise of the Network Society*, Oxford: Blackwell.
——(1997) *The Information Age: Economy, Society and Culture*, Vol. II, *The Power of Identity*, Oxford: Blackwell.
——(1998) *The Information Age: Economy, Society and Culture*, Vol. III, *End of Millennium*, Oxford: Blackwell.
Clegg, S. (1990) *Modern Organisations: Organizational Studies in the Post-Modern World*, London: Sage.
Cooper, R. (1992) 'Formal organization as representation: remote control, displacement and abbreviation', in M. Reed and M. Hughes, *Rethinking Organization: New Directions in Organizational Theory and Analysis*, London: Sage.

Crook, S., Pakulski, J. and Waters, M. (1992) *Postmodernization: Change in Advanced Society*, London: Sage.

Department of Health (DOH) (1989) *Working for Patients*, London: HMSO.

——(1992) *The Health of the Nation: A Strategy for Health in England*, London: HMSO.

——(1997) *The New NHS: Modern, Dependable*, London: The Stationery Office.

——(1998) *Our Healthier Nation: A Contract for Health*, London: The Stationery Office.

Dizard, W.P. (1989) *The Coming Information Age: An Overview of Technology, Economics, and Politics*, London: Longmans.

Featherstone, M. (1991) *Consumer Culture and Postmodernism*, London: Sage.

Fox, A. (1974) *Beyond Contract: Work, Power and Trust Relations*, London: Faber & Faber.

Fox, N. (1993) *Postmodernism, Sociology and Health*, Buckingham: Open University Press.

Fukuyama, F. (1996) *Trust: The Social Virtues and the Creation of Prosperity*, New York: The Free Press.

Gibson, W. (1984) *Neuromancer*, New York: Ace.

Goldthorpe, J.H., Lockwood, D., Bechhofer, F. and Platt, J. (1969) *The Affluent Worker in the Class Structure*, Cambridge: Cambridge University Press.

Harrison, B. (1994) *Lean and Mean: The Changing Landscape of Corporate Power in the Age of Flexibility*, New York: Basic Books.

Harvey, D. (1990) *The Condition of Postmodernity*, Oxford: Blackwell.

Held, D. (1995) *Democracy and the Global Order: From the Modern State to Cosmopolitan Governance*, Cambridge: Polity.

Heydebrand (1989) 'New organisational forms', *Work and Occupations* 16, 3: 323–57.

Hoggett, P. (1990) *Modernisation, Political Strategy and the Welfare State: An Organisational Perspective*, Studies in Decentralisation and Quasi-markets 2, Bristol: SAUS, University of Bristol.

——(1991) 'A new management in the public sector', *Policy & Politics*, 19, 4: 143–56.

——(1994) 'The politics of the modernisation of the UK welfare state', in R. Burrows and B. Loader (eds) *Towards a Post-Fordist Welfare State?*, London: Routledge.

Hurst, J. (1992) *The Reform of Health Care: A Comparative Analysis of Seven OECD Countries*, Paris: OECD.

Jessop, B. (1994) 'The transition to a Post-Fordist and Schumperterian workfare state', in R. Burrows and B. Loader (eds) *Towards a Post-Fordist Welfare State?*, London: Routledge.

Klein, R. (1995) *The New Politics of the NHS*, London: Longman.

Le Grand, J. (1990) 'Quasi-markets and social policy', July, School for Advanced Urban Studies, University of Bristol.

Loader, B.D. (1997) *The Governance of Cyberspace: Politics, Technology and Global Restructuring*, London: Routledge.

——(1998a) 'Welfare direct: informatics and the emergence of self-service welfare?', in J. Carter (ed.) *Postmodernity and the Fragmentation of Welfare*, London: Routledge.

——(1998b) *Cyberspace Divide: Equality, Agency and Policy in the Information Society*, London: Routledge.

McKeown, T. (1976) 'The modern rise of population and the role of medicine: dream, mirage or nemesis?', Rock Carling Monograph, London: Nuffield Provincial Hospitals Trust.

Marshall, G., Rose, D., Volgar, C. and Newby, H. (1985) 'Class, citizenship and distributional conflicts in modern Britain', *British Journal of Sociology* 36, 2: 259–84.

Moran, M. (1997) 'Explaining the rise of the market in health care', in W. Ranade (ed.) *Markets and Health Care: A Comparative Analysis*, London: Addison Wesley Longman.

Murray, R. (1991) 'The state after Henry', *Marxism Today*, May 22–7.

Navarro, V. (1986) *Crisis, Health and Medicine: A Social Critique*, London: Tavistock.

Negroponte, N. (1995) *Being Digital*, London: Hodder & Stoughton.

Petersen, A. and Lupton, D. (1996) *The New Public Health: Health and Self in the Age of Risk*, London: Sage.

Pollitt, C. (1990) *Managerialism and the Public Services*, Oxford: Blackwell.

Pyper, C. (1997) 'Trust me, I'm the patient', *The Wealth and Poverty of Networks: Tackling Social Exclusion*, Demos Collection, Issue 12: 41–3.

Reed, M. (1992) *The Sociology of Organizations: Themes, Perspectives and Prospects*, London: Harvester Wheatsheaf.

Reich, R. (1992) *The Work of Nations: Preparing Ourselves for the 21st Century*, New York: Vintage.

Saunders, P. (1984) 'Beyond housing classes: the sociological significance of private property rights in means of consumption', *International Journal of Urban and Regional Research* 8, 2: 202–27.

Stoker, G. (1989) 'Creating a local government for a Post-Fordist society: the Thatcherite project?', in J. Stewart and G. Stoker (eds) *The Future of Local Government*, Basingstoke: Macmillan.

Warde, A. (1994) 'Consumers, consumption and Post-Fordism', in R. Burrows and B. Loader (eds) *Towards a Post-Fordist Welfare State?*, London: Routledge.

Webster, F. and Robins, K. (1998) 'The iron cage of the information society', *Information, Communication & Society* 1, 1: 23–45.

Williams, F. (1989) *Social Policy: A Critical Introduction*, Cambridge: Polity.

——(1994) 'Social relations, welfare and the Post-Fordist debate', in R. Burrows and B. Loader (eds), *Towards a Post-Fordist Welfare State?*, London: Routledge.

Name index

Subject index